Towards a Positive Future

Towards a Positive Future

Stories, ideas and inspiration
from children with special educational needs,
their families and professionals

Janet O'Keefe (Editor)

J&R Press Ltd

© 2011 J&R Press Ltd

All rights reserved. No part of this publication may be reproduced, stored in a retrieval system or transmitted in any form or by any means, electronic, mechanical, photocopying, recording, scanning or otherwise, except under the terms of the Copyright Designs and Patents Act 1988 or under the terms of a licence issued by the Copyright Licensing Agency Ltd, without the permission in writing of the Publisher. Requests to the Publisher should be addressed to J&R Press Ltd, Farley Heath Cottage, Albury, Guildford GU5 9EW, or emailed to rachael_jrpress@btinternet.com.

The use of general descriptive names, registered names, trademarks, etc. in this publication does not imply, even in the absence of a specific statement, that such names are exempt from the relevant protective laws and regulations and therefore free for general use.

Library of Congress Cataloguing in Publication Data
British Library Cataloguing in Publication Data
A catalogue record for this book is available from the British Library
Cover design: Jim Wilkie
Project management, typesetting and design: J&R Publishing Services Ltd, Guildford, Surrey, UK; www.jr-publishingservices.co.uk

Printed and bound by CPI Group (UK) Ltd, Croydon, CR0 4YY

Contents

About the contributors vii
Foreword by Dr Hilary Gardner xii

Part I Background and Context

Chapter 1 Why me and why this book 1
Chapter 2 Setting the scene 9
Chapter 3 Finding support: Practical information for parents and expert witnesses 25

Part II Personal Stories

Chapter 4 Autism and Asperger syndrome: Communication, friendship and flexibility 35
Chapter 5 Behavioural, emotional and social conditions: Learning, feelings and mood 49
Chapter 6 Specific learning disability, dyslexia and dyscalculia: Reading, writing and calculating 59
Chapter 7 Speech, language and communication needs: Hearing, understanding and talking 71
Chapter 8 Learning disability: Mild, moderate, severe or complex 85

Part III The Future

Chapter 9 The long view: Disabled children become adults 97
Chapter 10 Celebrating strengths: The ordinariness of impairment 101
Chapter 11 Making it happen 109
Appendix 113
References and suggested reading 121
Glossary 127

About the contributors

Robert Ashton is a social entrepreneur, speaker and author. In common with many highly intelligent people, he was a shy, solitary child who did badly at school. His strong sense of justice and equality are rooted in his school days when he was misunderstood and overlooked. He has started and sold businesses, written 12 books and founded a successful charity. He is also a campaigner with a particular interest in mental health.

Susan Brooks is a chartered educational psychologist currently offering educational psychology services to a range of independent schools, FE and HE institutions in and around London and Hertfordshire. She also works as a consultant with Dyslexia Action. With over 18 years' experience in education, Susan has been employed by local education authorities as a teacher, special needs coordinator, educational psychologist and specialist educational psychologist. She has been a qualified teacher since 1991 and a qualified educational psychologist since 1997. Susan has worked in private practice since 2001. Between 2002 and 2009, she was employed as an Associate Lecturer in Developmental Psychology for the Open University.

Janet Farrugia qualified as a speech and language therapist in 1980 from University College London (UCL), and achieved a Masters Degree in Human Communication from City University in 2001. Janet has run an independent paediatric speech and language therapy practice since 1987, and in 1996 she opened Edenside Clinic, where she employs a team of eight speech and language therapists who provide therapy in local schools as well as in the purpose-designed clinic. Janet has contracts with local education authorities to provide speech and language therapy for children who have this provision on their Statements of Special Educational Need. Since 1996, she has also been involved in medico-legal work for Special Educational Needs Tribunals and has provided over 500 reports and attended as an expert witness at SENDIST on numerous occasions.

Hilary Gardner has been a speech and language therapist for over 30 years, working with children of all ages. She has provided a service in all types of settings; firstly in community and hospital paediatric clinics, then moving on to work in collaboration with education, in preschool and primary language units and then in an integrated 'language resourced' school. Alongside her clinical involvement, Hilary held lecturing and research posts at Birmingham, Manchester and Leeds Metropolitan Universities before arriving in Sheffield. She offers detailed assessment at the client's home or at a multidisciplinary clinic and also visits schools to advise on individual needs. Her expertise in the autistic spectrum relates to the moderate to higher end of the continuum, especially mainstream inclusion. As part of her work at Sheffield University, she has written on children's language disorders and screening in early years. Hilary has accredited medico-legal training and regularly works with case managers. She is the current Chair of the Association of Speech and Language Therapists in Independent Practice (ASLTIP).

Robert Love joined Christopher Davidson in 2011 and heads their dedicated education law team. Robert is a specialist in the law relating to special educational needs. His involvement in this area began as a result of successfully battling with his local education authority to get the right provision for his own son, who has special educational needs after suffering brain damage at birth. Robert became one of the first specialists in this area of the law and has been involved in many high-profile cases which have greatly improved the rights of parents of children with special educational needs. He continues to be a nationally renowned expert who is recognized by the *Good Lawyer Guide 2010* and by *Chambers and Partners Guide to the UK Legal Profession*. He is a member of the Advisory Board of the *Education and Public Law Journal* and is also a member of the Education Law Association.

Nicola Martin is currently the Director of Wellbeing and Disability Services at The London School of Economics where she takes a strategic lead in embedding disability equality into the culture of the organization. Nicola has particular expertise in working with students who identify with Asperger syndrome. She is an Honorary Visiting Fellow at the University of Cambridge, working with Professor Simon Baron-Cohen on a student voice project. Prior to the LSE appointment, she was a Principal Lecturer at Sheffield Hallam University, leading the Centre for Disability and Diversity Studies and The Autism Centre. Nicola is Senior Parliamentary Policy Adviser for The British Dyslexia Association, an Honorary Visiting Fellow at Sheffield Hallam University, and an external examiner for three Autism/Critical Disability Studies courses. In addition, she is a Visiting Professor at The Institute of Education in Hong Kong. Nicola has a very strong commitment to disability equality as a human rights issue and an important aspect of social justice. She has worked in education with disabled people across the age range continually since 1976, has four relevant degrees, a range of specialist qualifications and a string of publications which articulate a Social Model perspective on disability. Research interests include inclusive practice in further and higher education, emancipatory work with students who have Asperger syndrome, and disability activism and disablism in performing arts. She has lectured in Australia, New Zealand, USA, Europe and many UK universities. Nicola is Chair of The National Association of Disability Practitioners and Editor of *The Journal of Inclusive Practice in Further and Higher Education*.

Charlie Mead was the youngest headteacher in the West Midlands to run SEBD (Social, Emotional, and Behavioural Difficulties) schools for teenagers who been excluded from the mainstream system. Twenty-five years later, he is now a consultant child and educational psychologist, providing hands-on services to the National Autistic Society, mainstream academies and health and prison services on working effectively with students with complex needs – especially those with autism and challenging behaviour difficulties.

Janet O'Keefe qualified as a speech and language therapist in 1985 and from 1989 to 1997 was responsible for coordinating the paediatric services across West Suffolk. She has a special interest in children with autistic spectrum conditions, including Asperger syndrome, and for the last three years of her NHS employment she was the Mid Anglia Trust's specialist SLT for autism and hearing impairment. Janet is a member of the National Deaf Children's Society, an accreditation team member of the National Autistic Society, and is one of the honorary consultants in speech and language therapy for the Twins and Multiple Births Association (TAMBA). She was the RCSLT/ASLTIP Medico-Legal Representative from 1999–2002 and is a full member of the Expert Witness Institute. Currently, Janet undertakes approximately 80 independent speech and language therapy assessments and reports per year, submitted as part of statutory assessments for children with special educational needs or appeals to SENDIST. She also prepares expert reports for medico-legal cases in the High Court. She attends approximately 20 hearings a year as an expert witness. Janet's independent clinic, Wordswell, currently has contracts for speech and language therapy services for individual children with six local education authorities in the Eastern Region, and with individual families to see children in both state and independent schools. Recently, Janet founded The Clarity Foundation with Robert Ashton (see above).

Douglas Silas qualified as a solicitor in September 1997 and established Douglas Silas Solicitors in 2005. Prior to this, he trained and worked for over six years at Levenes Solicitors in the UK's first ever Education and Disability department, after which he established and headed a very successful Education and Public Law department for Alexander Harris Solicitors (now incorporated into Irwin Mitchell Solicitors). Douglas is also the current Honorary Legal Adviser to IPSEA (the Independent Panel for Special Educational Advice), which remains at the forefront of providing free, independent legal advice and support to parents of children with special needs. Over the years, Douglas has helped thousands of parents to get the right educational provision or placement for their child, even when they thought their case was hopeless. In sole practice, Douglas has successfully won or settled around 85% of cases during the past few years, the vast majority involving SEN appeals to the SEND Tribunal, as well as a number of Judicial Reviews and Statutory Appeals to the High Court against Tribunal decisions and local authorities.

Richard Soppitt is a consultant and Honorary Senior Lecturer in Child and Adolescent Psychiatry. He is approved under Section 12(2) of the 1983 Mental Health Act as having special expertise in the recognition of mental disorder. Richard works in a multi-agency team and specializes clinically in the diagnosis and management of neurodevelopmental disorders such as hyperkinetic (ADHD) and autistic spectrum conditions as well as emotional disorders such as depression and obsessive compulsive disorder. He has lectured nationally on autism and has also been featured in the January–February 2007 edition of *SEN Magazine* discussing autism in the 21st century, and in the March/April edition discussing ADHD. He is contributing a chapter on ADHD in a forthcoming book edited by Peer and Reid (2011) and recently published an audit on ADHD treatment and NICE guidelines.

Lidia Trojanowska started in the field of autism 12 years ago and, coming from an academic background, it soon became apparent to her that ABA (Applied Behaviour Analysis) was so much more than the research she had read about. Training under consultants from the UK and USA, she advanced from School Shadow to Learning Support Assistant, Tutor to Senior Tutor, and from Lead Tutor to Supervisor, which has given her insight into every level of ABA service delivery. She has worked with LEAs, schools and private individuals, both in the UK and internationally. Her work in the Middle East as a school psychologist, assessment coordinator and special needs and mainstream teacher, further developed her skill-set of primary school-aged children. Working in the USA at a residential school and as an ABA programme manager allowed her to gain invaluable experience with both secondary school-aged children and young adults developing self help and vocational skills. As the Director of Omega AIT Ltd, Lidia supervises ABA Home Programmes and trains tutors.

Louise Wilkinson is Training Manager at the charity Child Brain Injury Trust; her role is to raise awareness about the issues that children, young people and their families face following the devastation of childhood acquired brain injury. She has trained over 2000 professionals across education, healthcare, social services and, more recently, those working with young offenders and those at risk of offending. Louise has also spoken at many conferences on this subject including SEN, Youth Offending and ABI conferences. Since joining the Child Brain Injury Trust in 2008, Louise's passion for ensuring that these children and young people receive the appropriate support to enable them to achieve their full potential in life has helped raise the profile of this hidden disability.

Clive Yeadon is an independent social welfare and social policy consultant and independent social worker. Clive has been through the ranks in the field of social work. Now as an independent consultant, he is in great demand as a 'problem solver' in complex cases. His education law qualifications put him in the somewhat rare position of understanding the inter-relationship of social services and education legislation, and his breadth of experience means that his work as a witness at SEN Tribunals can be very important, especially where parents are seeking a residential school placement.

Foreword

This book describes the present legal process for establishing an adequate educational 'statement' of the needs of a child with a disability, or appealing against one that is deemed to be inadequate. The editor has gathered together parental accounts of their experiences of that process and these form the main body of the book. It does not make an entirely easy read emotionally. Some of the stories are raw in the telling but in sum form a tribute to all the parents and professionals who have dedicated themselves to enhancing children's prospects without compromise.

This book forms the precursor to a weightier volume which will be written when radical reform of the present special needs education legislation (in England) has been settled. The road to the point where reform has been acknowledged as necessary has sometimes been rocky. The present legislation, although working well for many, has caused anguish for some parents as they saw their child's needs go unrecognized or compromised by provision that did not suit them. They have had to fight their way through a lengthy and complex process to gain the right level of provision for their child, sometimes supported by expert professionals, sometimes alone.

In producing this book, the editor and her team hope that we can learn from experience and, despite the present economic challenge, move towards a system that is workable and honest in its ambition. We can all (both parent and professional) contribute towards that positive future by making our voices heard, telling it as it is and saying how it should be.

Dr Hilary Gardner
Department of Human Communication Sciences
The University of Sheffield
September 2011

Part I
Background and Context

1 Why me and why this book

Introduction

When I qualified as a speech and language therapist (SALT) from the Central School of Speech and Drama in 1985, I could not possibly have imagined what life would have in store. As many of you who watched or read *The King's Speech* this year will know, speech therapy grew out of actors working with wounded soldiers from the First World War. However, sharing training with drama students and teachers no longer fits the funding model, although it makes perfect sense, and even though it was a forward thinking degree course with great lecturers, it has been a casualty of university cuts and reorganizations and no longer exists.

Like all new graduates at that time, we assumed that we would get a job in the NHS and, although we might change jobs to gain promotion or to specialize, we would always be employed by the NHS. I was very lucky that I got my first job even before I qualified, so that I started paid employment immediately. I had a mixed post working with both children and adults alongside senior and specialist therapists, many of whom are my professional mentors today. I loved my chosen career and could see that what I did made a difference to the quality of life of the people and families with whom I worked.

I met my future husband, moved to East Anglia, got married, gained promotion to become a Chief Speech and Language Therapist for Paediatrics and Learning Disabilities and was inspired by a consultant community paediatrician. Together, we were part of a multidisciplinary team that designed and oversaw the building of our very own Child Development Centre. Together, we developed ways of truly working together to not only assess and diagnose but also treat and support children and their families. This included providing social skills groups to youngsters with an autistic spectrum condition (ASC) who weren't yet in crisis but whom we knew would not get through their adolescence without strategies in place to avoid the mental health issues suffered by their predecessors. I enjoyed everything about my job and loved every client group – particularly the more complex and challenging ones. Then the recession of the early 1990s hit and accountants took over the NHS. All the professional heads of service were made redundant across East Anglia to be replaced by General or Locality Managers. So in one fell swoop I lost my professional support and supervision and also my career progression. The Health Authority was split between purchasers and providers, and the providers were split into different Trusts for Community vs. Acute Hospital Services; Adult Mental Health Services were split off too. I quickly became disillusioned by being told whom I could see, when and for how long I could see them, which was not based on patient need but on NHS resources. 'They' were more interested in how many patients I saw in a day rather than whether what I did with them enabled them to progress or not. In fact, if they were discharged and were re-referred, they could be counted again!

I had my first baby but returning part-time at the same grade was made very difficult. The Trust did not like flexible hours of working and did not really like part-timers at all. I was running around 'putting sticking plasters' on things and not doing anything properly. I imagined the families of my patients saying, 'The speech and language therapist is very nice but we only see her once in a blue moon, so what she does doesn't make a difference.' In my eyes, if I was not making a difference, the job was not worth doing. I sought mentors from outside the Trust and discovered Neuro-Linguistic Programming. During my Master Practitioner Programme, I was introduced to exemplars of excellence from many different walks of life, such as Frank Farrelly, Raymond Blanc and Brian Keenan.

Frank Farrelly has gained international recognition as a profoundly gifted therapist. He is the author of several publications, including *Provocative Therapy* (with Jeff Brandsma). He has presented numerous workshops, seminars and demonstrations of his work for professional audiences throughout the United States, Europe and Australasia. His expertise in working with severely disturbed clients makes him an especially interesting and important teacher. Provocative Therapy was developed in an inpatient ward as Frank, dissatisfied with his effectiveness as a psychotherapist, began to explore new procedures for promoting significant, resilient change in chronic and recalcitrant patients. He worked in this institutional setting for 17 years, continuing to develop and refine his techniques. Frank said, 'If you enjoy what you are doing, you are in great danger of becoming good at it.' I believe the converse is also true. If you don't enjoy what you are doing, then you are in great danger of being lousy at it! You may continue to be competent but not excellent and inspirational, and I wanted to strive for excellence.

Raymond Blanc is now one of the most renowned chefs in the UK. He has earned Michelin stars and an OBE but is totally self taught. Raymond said,

'When something is right you just know it inside deep in your gut.' I knew that what I was doing in the NHS did not feel right, for me or for those people with whom I worked.

Brian Keenan was an unknown university lecturer from Belfast when, in April 1986, he was taken hostage in Lebanon for almost five years. His book, *An Evil Cradling*, was hard to read but taught me not to be afraid to be myself. Brian told me to 'choose joy'.

By the time I had finished my Master Practitioner Course, I had handed in my notice. It was scary to think that I might be stacking shelves in a supermarket by Christmas. I wrote to Brian, and he helped me to name my new business and my clinic building 'Wordswell'. So in 1997 I started Wordswell, an independent speech and language therapy clinic, and have met many inspirational families and children, every one of whom has taught me about individual differences, how children learn and how to communicate better.

Working with children with special educational needs and supporting parents

From 1998, I undertook assessments and wrote reports to be used in Statutory Assessments and Appeals to the Special Educational Needs Tribunal. From 1999, I went with parents as an expert witness to give live oral evidence. I was again fortunate that the Association of Speech and Language Therapists in Independent Practice (ASLTIP) had been born and had started providing medico-legal training. I became the representative on the ASLTIP Executive responsible for medico-legal matters, ran the courses and manned the jointly funded ASLTIP/RCSLT Medico-Legal Helpline for the profession until 2002.

I gained insight into the appeal process itself, as well as the emotional stress it causes parents, through working with education law expert solicitors, barristers, lay representatives, charities and support groups, as well as excellent specialist independent schools, other experts from related fields such as educational psychology, occupational therapy, audiology, psychiatry and, of course, parents themselves. Through working as a SALT with these families, I know that it is very difficult practically, financially and emotionally having a child with special needs. Many parents suffer worry and guilt about getting a diagnosis for the child they have created and brought into the world. The lack of sleep, lack of support and lack of insight from friends and family, however caring, is hard and stressful. It is not easy for parents to find the right people to talk to in order to acquire the information they need about their child's condition, what treatments are available and how to access or get funding for them. Everyone seems to have their own agenda for what they tell parents based on who employs them and what resources are available locally. Parents become frustrated and feel patronized when 'professionals', who do not know their child or who have spent five minutes with them, label them and try to determine their future. Parents are supposed to be grateful when they get an appointment to see someone, however infrequent and inconvenient it is, because the professionals are doing their best in difficult circumstances. It is rare to see the same person twice. Everyone assesses and advises but few actually do anything to help the child from either the child or the family's perspective. They are ticking their boxes and covering their backs. What they are not doing is putting the needs of the child first. It is frustrating for parents who know their child to have their views dismissed because they are 'just the parent'.

You may ask how I describe this from the heart when I am just a SALT. It is because I thought I knew the system well enough that my husband and I fostered a child who has a major medical condition, special educational and social, emotional and behavioural needs. We thought it would be easier for us as we had chosen to care for this child with our eyes open. However, it has been the hardest part of the journey so far, as my experience and expertise have made absolutely no difference to how we and the child we care for have been treated by the statutory services. The difference, maybe, is that I have a network of experts and education and family lawyers who can help and support us, but it is difficult to mix business with friendship and impose on and ask too much of colleagues. The charities, parent support groups and pro bono lawyers are brilliant, if you can find them. It is an unfair system, even for me. The Legal Aid lawyers are brilliant, but if you own your own house you cannot qualify and it looks probable that Legal Help will be phased out for special educational needs cases completely.

Over the last 14 years, I have undertaken hundreds of detailed assessments and written reports on children and adults from all over the country. These have been submitted to support Statutory Assessment or an Appeal to the Special Educational Needs Tribunal or to court in medico-legal cases. I have attended over 100 hearings to give live oral evidence and be cross-examined. I am not diagnosing or recommending anything different to what I was while employed by the NHS, but the difference is that I am now listened to and my evidence has influenced practice. It matters how and where children with special educational needs are educated. It matters how they are supported. Many need integrated therapy in an educational context where teaching informs therapy and therapy informs teaching, not bolt-on provision in a school which is either unsupportive, unsupported, inexperienced, or all three. There are some good state schools with excellent heads and SENCOs, and where integration and inclusion can and does work for some children. The problem is, if done properly it is not a cheap option, and we are in a culture of cuts.

Purpose of this book

First, may I make it clear that I know many children with SEN and their families are happy with the way they have been supported by the system and all the professionals working with them. This book is not intended to disparage committed and hardworking professionals, but rather to highlight the stories of real children and how attitudes and procedures could have been improved to relieve them and their families of stress and anguish, giving us lessons to learn as we enter a period of change.

This book is written from the perspective of an expert witness speech and language therapist, but also of a parent/carer. It comprises fifteen personal stories from some of the families that I or my colleagues have worked with over the last 15 years, and the effect that going through the SEN system and the process of appeal has had on their lives. Governments monitor the outcomes of the processes but not the emotional impact, nor the stress, nor even the educational outcome. Through these stories, I hope to answer some of the common questions asked of me by parents and professional colleagues, and illustrate some of the things I have learned which I hope will help both in the future. I will try to focus on what we know works and how this can continue to work – whatever the future political or legal system we find ourselves under in the coming months or years. The Big Society is a mind shift for many of us, but by working together and networking we can continue to make a positive difference to all those we come into contact with on a daily basis.

So how can this book be as useful as possible to both parents and professional colleagues living and working with children with special educational needs?

It will, hopefully, give answers to some of the questions that I am frequently asked. Chapter 2 outlines the current procedures to do with the process of appeal. Chapter 3 covers many of the issues that parents and professionals need to know when they live and work with a child with SEN:

- How do you find people to advocate or represent or support you in order to get an assessment?

- How do you access independent experts?
- What is the difference between professional and expert opinion?
- How do you use that information to get the child the support services they need in school?
- What are tribunals like?
- How do you prepare for a tribunal hearing? Although at the time of writing we don't yet know the final outcome of the current health, education and social care reforms, it looks likely that there will remain a tribunal system to which parents can appeal.

The following chapters feature case studies and look at families with children of various ages with different types of SEN. Broadly speaking, they have needs that fall into one of the following categories:

- Autistic Spectrum Condition, including Asperger syndrome;
- Behavioural, Emotional and Social Conditions (BESC), including ADHD;
- Specific Learning Disability (dyslexia);
- Speech, Language and Communication Needs (SLCN), including hearing disability/deafness;
- Moderate or Severe Learning Disability/Complex Needs, including physical disability.

However, children whose cases go to appeal at tribunal are rarely straightforward, and often fall into more than one of these groups.

Some of these stories have happy endings and some do not. Some are still on their journey. Some of the children have attended mainstream school with support, and others have needed to attend a unit or specialist school. Some families have been able to afford specialist legal support from solicitors and barristers, and others have represented themselves or been represented by charities or other lay representatives. What they all have in common is that the whole process has taken its toll on the family emotionally, practically and financially. All that they want is for their children's needs to be recognized and for their children to reach their potential, whatever that potential is, so that they have a greater chance of being independent in the future and thereby not becoming a greater burden on society.

This is not designed to be an academic book, nor can I claim that it is representative of everyone's experiences. The families that commission independent reports from me and my expert witness colleagues are already on the road to appeal. There are many families who are getting good assessments, reports and support from their local team and they don't phone me up to tell me. This is a collection of real stories and experiences from which we can learn. We can learn from what has gone right for children and families, and we can learn from what has not gone well and aim to do things differently in the future.

The final chapters bring together all the learning points, discuss what disability is and how parents and professionals can work together to share skills, knowledge and expertise, and to support children with SEN to achieve their potential both academically and socially and how we can individually and collectively contribute to 'The Big Society'.

Concluding remarks

Although I have endeavoured to make this book as comprehensive as possible, it is not possible to cover every topic and I apologise in advance for any omissions. The inspiration for this book has been Rachael Wilkie, a truly supportive publisher, and the many families of children with SEN.

Children and their families are anonymized for confidentiality and neither have I identified which professional contributors have collaborated for each chapter specifically to ensure equality of acknowledgment with parents. All references and further suggested reading are listed together at the end of the book.

Although the identities are disguised, the personal stories are all real.

2 Setting the scene

Introduction

This chapter is historical in as much as it sets out the process of identifying, assessing and appealing statements of special educational needs (SEN) at the time of writing even though we know this system is likely to change imminently. However, it is helpful to put all the personal stories into context.

The current SEN Code of Practice came out in 2001. This provides practical advice to local education authorities (LEAs), maintained schools, early years settings and others on carrying out their statutory duties to identify, assess and make provision for children's special educational needs. It outlines the different processes that need to take place and the responsibilities each agency has for meeting each child's needs. The SEN Code of Practice has the status of 'statutory guidance' which means that all agencies involved, including health and social services, must have regard to the Code – they must not ignore it.

School Action/Early Years Action

When an education practitioner who works daily with the child or SENCO (in the case of a pre-school child), or a class teacher or SENCO (in the case of a school-aged child), identifies a child with SEN, they should devise interventions that are additional to or different from those provided as part of the setting's usual curriculum offer and strategies (paras 4.20 and 5.43 of the Code of Practice). (Note: for brevity the term 'school' is used from now on to cover all types of educational and early years settings.) A trigger for intervention could be concern (by a parent or professional) about a child who, despite receiving appropriate early education/differentiated learning opportunities:

- makes little or no progress even when teaching approaches are particularly targeted;
- shows signs of difficulty in developing literacy or mathematics skills which result in poor attainment in some curriculum areas;
- continues to work at levels significantly below those expected for peers of a similar age in certain areas;

- presents persistent emotional and/or behavioral difficulties, not ameliorated by the behaviour management techniques being used;
- has sensory or physical problems and makes little or no progress despite provision of personal aids and equipment;
- has communication and/or interaction difficulties and requires specific individual interventions in order to access learning (paras 4.21 and 5.44 of the Code of Practice).

Action should then be taken from within the school's resources to enable the child to learn and progress to the maximum possible. This may involve action such as: the deployment of extra staff; provision of different learning materials or special equipment; introduction to some group/individual support; and staff development and training to introduce more effective strategies.

An Individual Education Plan should be devised detailing strategies to enable the child to progress and 3–4 SMART targets (Specific, Measurable, Achievable, Relevant and Time Bound) should be given. For example: 'To be able to understand the concept of "after" in relation to a sequence of events, on 9 out of 10 occasions by the end of June'.

The early years setting or school has a duty to inform parents that special educational provision is being made for their child because they have identified the child as having SEN.

School Action Plus/Early Years Action Plus

This is characterized by the involvement of external support services and is actioned when School Action has resulted in little or no progress in specific areas over a long period of time. It is likely to follow a decision taken by the SENCO and colleagues in consultation with parents at a meeting to review the IEP. The external services can help: through advice on IEPs and targets; more specialized assessments; support for specialist strategies or materials; and sometimes providing support for particular activities.

For example, if the child has speech, language or communication difficulties that are causing significant barriers to learning so that s/he is struggling to access the curriculum, then a decision is made to request help from external agencies. In this case, it would be most appropriate to contact a speech and language therapist, who would observe and assess the child and be able to advise the school on new IEP targets, approaches and strategies to help. Parental consent must be sought and received before a child is seen by an external agency.

Request for Statutory Assessment Procedure

Requests for a statutory assessment can be made by parents or by the child's school or setting. Health services and social service departments can also draw children to the LEA's attention. (This is particularly likely to happen with children under 5 with complex needs who are not yet attending school but may be in an early education setting.)

If a school concludes that, despite all the interventions and strategies they have been trying so far, the child's needs are so substantial that they cannot be effectively met within the resources normally available to the school, and the child has demonstrated significant cause for concern, then a request can be made to the LEA to carry out a statutory assessment. Schools must consult with parents before requesting a statutory assessment. Before the decision is made whether or not to make an assessment, the LEA must write to parents, setting out the procedures to follow, explaining time limits, encouraging parents to provide their own evidence, etc.

Parents can make a request for a statutory assessment to the LEA at any time, independently of the school, if they believe that their child has special educational needs that are preventing them from progressing sufficiently and the school is unable to provide the necessary level of help. However, it is advisable that parents discuss this with the school, because the staff will be familiar with the range of evidence the LEA needs to see before making a decision. It is in the child's best interests that the school and parents are able to work together on any request for a statutory assessment. If the request is made by the parents, the LEA must contact them to find out more about their concerns and their current involvement with their child's special educational provision. They must also contact the school to advise them that a request has been made and ask them for the type of evidence outlined in the section below.

Parents should also be informed about the local parent partnership services, which provide information about other sources of independent advice such as local or national voluntary organizations, and any local support group that may be able to help them. Parents are told that they can provide any private advice or opinion and that this advice will be taken into account.

LEAs need to examine a wide range of evidence to assess whether or not a statutory assessment will be carried out, including reviewing the school's assessment of the child's needs, gathering input from a range of professionals such as educational psychologists, support teachers and others, and looking at what action the school has taken to meet those needs. The LEA will also ask for evidence of the child's levels of academic attainment and rates of progess in the context of attainment of their peers, their own rate of progress over time, and expectations of their performance (para 7.34 of the Code of Practice).

Most children with special educational needs have strengths and difficulties in one, some or all of the areas of speech, language and communication, and their communication needs may be diverse and complex. However, if the LEA considers that there are teaching programmes which could be provided for the child in school in collaboration with the LEA or external support services, then it may conclude that intervention should be provided at School Action Plus and that reassessment is not necessary (Para 7:55 of the Code of Practice).

Whether the LEA grants or turns down the request for assessment, it must write to the parents and the school within six weeks, explaining the reasons behind the decision. If they turn down the request, they must describe the provision that they consider is appropriate to meet the child's needs and inform parents of their right to appeal to the SEN and Disability Tribunal (SEND Tribunal), the time limits for an appeal and the availability and details of a local Disagreement Resolution Service.

If the request for a statutory assessment is granted, the LEA will then seek advice. This should be done immediately the decision has been made. All those from whom advice is requested are asked to respond within six weeks. The advice sought is demarcated into five sections as follows and advice is sought from relevant professionals within these categories:

- parental advice
- educational advice (from schools and teachers)
- medical advice (from doctors, speech and language therapists, occupational therapists and physiotherapists)
- psychological advice (from educational or clinical psychologists)
- Social Services advice

The response can be as short as one line saying, 'Not known to this service', or a full detailed report.

Parents are entitled to provide their own reports from experts as part of the statutory assessment procedure. Many LEAs give clear parental guidelines as to the sort of information required and give headings/questions for parents to respond to. Parents should also be given the name of an LEA officer from whom they can request information and to whom their advice must be sent.

The LEA also gives guidance to the other agencies from whom advice is sought about the parameters of the advice they should give, as guided by the Code of Practice. Parents must be informed by the LEA that their child may be assessed by a range of professionals. They have the right to know when this will happen, who will be carrying it out and for what purpose. Parents are allowed to be present at any assessment or interview. However, the appropriateness of this should be discussed.

The LEA must also seek the views of the child or young person in question as part of the statutory assessment procedure. This is not always appropriate or possible, depending on the age and circumstances of the child or young person. However, the methods that can be used, such as an Advocate, should be discussed and agreed by all parties to establish the most effective way for a child's views to be heard.

Statement of Special Educational Needs

All the necessary advice should be received within six weeks of it being requested. It is then used as the basis for the decision that the LEA has to make as to whether it is necessary to produce a Statement in order for the child's special educational needs to be met. The LEA will produce a Statement only when it considers that the provision necessary to meet the child's needs cannot reasonably be provided within the resources normally available to mainstream schools in the area. The Code of Practice outlines a framework to support that decision-making process but allows for local interpretation which reflects the range of the local provision and the funding arrangements.

Each LEA should provide information which sets out the provision that it expects normally to be met from maintained schools' budget shares and that element of such provision that the authority expect normally to be met by the authority from funds which it holds centrally. The situation has been further complicated with the introduction of Academies and Free Schools, which have the legal status of independent schools. Parents are advised to check the latest information from the charities and helplines listed in the Appendix.

If the LEA decides not to produce a Statement of Special Educational Needs it must notify the parents telling them this and the reasons for it within two weeks after the statutory assessment process has been completed. It should also make sure that the child's parents are fully aware of the provision that is available within the school to meet the child's special educational needs.

The statutory assessment process will culminate in a significant amount of information being written and shared about a child's special educational needs. The LEA might decide to issue a 'Note in Lieu of the Statement', which should set out the reasons for the LEA's decision not to produce a Statement and the supporting evidence. It is good practice for some further opportunity for discussion and explanation to be offered.

At the same time as parents are informed that the LEA will not produce a Statement, they must also be informed of their right to appeal to the SEND Tribunal, the time limits for this appeal and the availability of parent partnership and disagreement resolution services.

Proposed and Final Statements

If the LEA decides to produce a Statement of Special Educational Needs it must first draft a Proposed Statement. This is complete in Part 2: Description of the child's needs, and Part 3: Provision to meet these needs, but Part 4: School placement, is left blank until the Final Statement is issued. This Proposed Statement must be sent to the child's parents within two weeks of the completion of the statutory assessment process.

If the parents feel that Part 2 represents an accurate description of their child's needs and that Part 3 sets out appropriate provision to meet their child's needs, then a Final Statement can be issued without amendments. However, if they are unhappy with the way their child's needs have been described or the provision that has been outlined, then they have 15 days to contact the LEA and request a meeting to discuss the contents of the Statement. Following the meeting, they have a further 15 days to make representations or request more meetings. Following the final meeting the parents have 15 days to make further comments to the LEA. The LEA must then send a copy of the Final Statement to the child's parents, with the named school written in Part 4. All the advice received by the LEA which has been taken into consideration during the statutory assessment process must be attached as Appendices. The whole process, from the initial request for a statutory assessment to the issuing of the Final Statement, should be completed within six months.

A Statement is a legally binding document that describes a child's special educational needs, what sort of provision must be made by the school and LEA in meeting those needs and where it should happen. An LEA school or setting cannot ignore the contents of the Statement; the child is entitled to the provision that is described.

If parents disagree with the Final Statement, they have the right to appeal if:

(a) their concerns with the Proposed Statement in relation to Parts 2 and/or 3 were not addressed;

(b) they disagree with the school named in Part 4 as they do not believe it can meet their child's special educational needs.

Parents need to be aware that a Statement of Special Educational Needs is a legal document. Provision specified in a Statement must be provided and, if the school cannot make the necessary provision then the local authority is under a legal obligation to 'arrange' the provision. The effectiveness of a Statement depends on achieving the full identification of the child's special educational needs in Part 2 with quantified and specified provision in Part 3 (including, for example, number of hours per week of TA support, specified input from a specialist teacher or amount of input per week from a qualifed speech and language therapist/occupational therapist). Achieving effective Statements will depend on the reports submitted as part of the statutory assessment process. In some cases, it is necessary for parents to seek additional assessments and reports from independent professionals.

SEND Tribunal

If parents are not able to reach agreement with the LEA about their child's special educational needs, they may be able to appeal to SEND Tribunal. There is a two month time limit for appealing which starts from the date on the LEA's letter giving their final written decision. SEND Tribunal is a free service which can also make a contribution towards expenses in attending the Tribunal hearing, such as travel costs. Currently, appeals to SEND tribunal follow the following format:

1. Appeal – week 0

2. LEA response – week 6

3. SO1 from the LEA – week 6

4. Applications by either party for varying SEN directions – week 6

5. SO1 from parents – week 9

6. All information to tribunal and other party – week 16

7. Final working document – week 18

8. Final hearing – week 20

9. Decision – week 22

Appeals to SEND Tribunals can be lodged if the LEA:

- will not carry out a statutory assessment of a child's special educational needs, following a request by parents or by the child's school;
- refuses to make a Statement of a child's special educational needs, following a statutory assessment;
- refuses to reassess a child's special educational needs (following a request by parents or by the child's school) if a new assessment has not been made for at least six months;
- decides not to maintain a child's Statement;
- decides not to change the Statement after reassessing a child;
- has made a Statement, or has changed a previous Statement, and parents disagree with the content of any of the parts.
- From 2010, a new right of appeal was introduced. Parents now have a right of appeal if the LEA decides not to amend the Statement following an annual review.

Parents cannot appeal to SEND Tribunal if they are unhappy about:

- the way the LEA carried out the assessment, or the length of time that it took;
- how the LEA or the school is arranging to provide the help set out in their child's Statement;
- the way the school is meeting their child's needs at School Action or School Action Plus;

Parents also cannot appeal because they want 'the best' education for their child. For example, if they believe School A is better than School B, they cannot appeal against School B just on this basis, unless School B cannot provide appropriate provision to meet their child's needs whereas school A can.

The appeal process

The appeal process is complex. Information and advice on the process are available from the SEND website (www.sendist.gov.uk) as well as charities that specialize in providing support to parents through the appeal process (see list in the Appendix).

Parents must appeal within two months of the date on the letter from the LEA giving their decision. If parents are outside the time frame, they can ask for an extension, which may be granted if there are extenuating circumstances that have prevented them from lodging their appeal in time. SEN appeals of all types have standard directions issued at the time they are registered, called SEN Appeal Directions.

Parents need to explain the decision against which they are appealing and give the reasons why they are appealing and what they are asking the tribunal to do. These are the basis for the 'grounds of appeal'. Parents should attach all information and any evidence that supports their appeal.

Once the appeal has been sent in, it is registered within 10 working days of its receipt. At this point, the 20-week timeline begins. SEND Tribunal will inform parents that their appeal has been registered and will also inform them of the date their appeal will be heard – 20 weeks later. At the same time, a Case Directions Form and an Attendance Form are sent stating the dates by which all information to be considered at the hearing must be received by SEND Tribunal. It also states when SEND Tribunal needs to be informed about the witnesses (if any) and anyone else who will be attending the hearing.

Parents need to think very carefully about which witnesses they should bring to a hearing. This decision-making process is helped by any reports written by expert witnesses on the child, as these help to highlight the child's key areas of need in relation to outstanding disputes between parents and the LEA. Parents can bring three witnesses or, with permission from SEND Tribunal, four if it is felt that this will help the tribunal reach a decision. A typical selection of witnesses might be: an educational psychologist; the head teacher from the proposed school parents want named in Part 4 of the Statement, and possibly a teacher who can talk about how the child is coping currently in school; and/or a speech and language therapist, an occupational therapist or physiotherapist (depending on whether the child has needs in these areas).

Once the appeal has been registered a copy is sent to the LEA. They will also be sent a Case Directions and an Attendance Form. The LEA has to respond within 30 working days of being sent the parents' appeal notice. It will send a copy of its response and any accompanying documents to SEND Tribunal and to the parents. The LEA will have the same timetable as parents to send further information and evidence to SEND Tribunal.

The LEA's response must say whether or not they oppose the parental appeal and, if so, why. They should provide a summary of the facts and, whenever possible, they must inform SEND Tribunal what the child involved thinks about the issues. The LEA may also contact parents about the appeal as, having looked at the evidence again, they might feel that they can provide some or all of what is requested.

Parents should try to send in all their documents with their appeal. The Case Directions will explain if other documents can be sent and by when. Parents and the LEA are required to provide information on the Further Information Form (SO1) about the areas of disagreement, or any additional information they intend to provide, their representatives, witnesses and others appearing at the final hearing. The LEA must submit this form by week 6 and the parents must submit it by week 9. The SEN Appeal Directions will require all further evidence to be provided to the tribunal and the other party by week 16.

At week 16, a team within the administration reviews all cases. Each case is looked at to see if there is anything outstanding which might prevent it from proceeding to the final hearing. In such circumstances, the case is placed before a tribunal judge to decide what action should be taken.

At week 18 a Final Working Document should be submitted by the LEA, with the objective that parents respond with areas of agreement and disagreement.

Changing or withdrawing the appeal

Any changes to the appeal, including a request to withdraw, must be made in writing on a 'request for changes' form from SEND Tribunal, which is available on the website (www.sendist.gov.uk). The amendments sought and the reasons for the amendments must be set out on the form, a copy of which must also be sent to the LEA.

Appeals can only be withdrawn with consent from SEND Tribunal. If this happens more than 10 working days before the hearing, then consent is normally given. If a request to withdraw is sent less than 10 working days before the hearing, it is necessary to explain why this has happened so close to the hearing. This request is considered by a tribunal judge who will decide what further action, if any, should be taken.

The hearing

A DVD is available on request that gives some idea of what happens at a hearing. Hearings are fixed for a certain time and parents and the LEA are asked to arrive 30 minutes before the start time in order to meet the clerk, and ask any questions. Sometimes last-minute agreements or amendments may be made to the Working Document before the hearing starts. New evidence should not normally be brought to the hearing by either party. If additional evidence is felt to be important then applications will need to be made on the 'request for changes' form. Permission may or may not be given, depending on the reasons given and the timescales.

Hearings take place at various Tribunal Service buildings up and down the country, if possible within 90 minutes of where the parents live. In special circumstances, a hearing may take place in a hotel. The length of each hearing depends on the contents of the appeal and the number of witnesses attending.

Appeals are heard by a panel of three tribunal members: the Chair, who is a legally qualified tribunal judge, and two specialist members who have been appointed because of their knowledge and experience of children with special educational needs and disabilities.

Parents do not have to attend the hearing, although it is beneficial to do so. The panel will want to hear anything parents have to say about their child in relation to his/her current situation. They do not want to hear what is contained in the papers or about procedural problems. Parents may also want to ask questions of the LA and any witnesses they may bring. Parents can nominate (or appoint) someone to represent them at the hearing, whether or not they attend. Solicitors or barristers can represent parents but they have to be funded by the parents as there is no public (or Legal Help) funding for this. The child in question can attend the hearing and give evidence, if appropriate, and the child wants to do so. However, it is unlikely that they will stay for the full hearing so arrangements to take them home or out of the building need to be made.

Another person can be brought to the hearing for parental support but they will not be allowed to take part, and their name must also be on the

Attendance Form. Because it is a private hearing, tribunals will not agree to let other people attend except parent supporters or possibly trainee barristers or solicitors.

Often, a report by a professional who has assessed the child will contain all the information that the tribunal panel needs to consider, so it may not be necessary for that person to attend the hearing in person. If parents have asked a witness to attend who is unhappy about doing so, parents can write to the tribunal and request a witness summons at least 15 working days before the hearing, explaining why they feel it is important for the witness to attend. If the tribunal agrees, they will issue a witness summons for parents to give to the witness, who will then have to attend the hearing unless there are very good extenuating circumstances.

Parents have the chance to ask questions of the LA and the witnesses and also add anything they consider is important but has not been mentioned. Parents, witnesses and somebody who attends the hearing specifically to look after the child can claim travel expenses for public transport or mileage for cars. Taxis should only be used in exceptional circumstances and must be authorized in advance. Witnesses can also claim a fixed amount for loss of earnings.

The decision

The decision and reasons should be received by post within 10 working days of the hearing, although often it is longer than this. The decision will be posted to both parties. A leaflet is also sent setting out in detail various options, which include the following:

- When parents have received a decision from the tribunal that they consider to be wrong on a point of law or that there is another reason why the tribunal should look again at its decision, parents can appeal to the Administrative Appeals Chamber of the Upper Tribunal but they must first apply to the SEND Tribunal for permission to appeal.

When the appeal has been decided, the LEA must comply with the SEND Tribunal's decision beginning with the date the decision was issued, as follows:

- To start the assessment or reassessment process – 4 weeks
- To make a Statement – 5 weeks
- To change a Statement – 5 weeks

- To change the school named in line with parents' wishes – 2 weeks
- To continue a Statement – immediately
- To cancel (cease to maintain) a Statement – immediately

These timescales also apply when the LEA does not oppose the appeal.

If the LEA does not comply with the order within the specified time, parents may have to apply to the High Court to enforce it. They can also make a complaint to the Local Government Ombudsman by contacting the Advice Team or by writing to the Local Government Ombudsman (see Appendix for details).

Maintaining a Statement and the annual review

Each Statement must be reviewed annually and the Code of Practice sets out a framework of how this should take place, so that most Annual Review Reports follow a very similar format.

Prior to the annual review, all professionals working with the child and parents submit a report. This should include recent assessment scores such as National Curriculum levels, reading and spelling levels and results from standardized assessments carried out by professionals such as educational psychologists and speech and language therapists. Progress should be monitored in relation to targets that have been worked on in relation to objectives in the Statement.

An annual review should include a meeting between parents and key professionals working with the child. This may involve teachers, educational psychologists, speech and language therapists, occupational therapists, etc. Views are taken from both the parents and the child. Recommendations can be made to the LEA for amendments to the Statement.

Future objectives relating to the objectives in Part 3 of the Statement should be identified through the annual review process for the forthcoming year. Short-term targets should be set to meet these annual review objectives. These should be reviewed regularly and preferably, on at least a termly basis.

Ceasing to maintain a Statement

The LEA can decide not to maintain a child's Statement if they think it is no longer necessary. They can only make this decision after close consultation with the parents. If the LEA decides that a child's Statement is no longer necessary, it must write and tell the parents, giving its reasons, and provide copies of any evidence it has used to support its decision.

Parents have the right to appeal against this decision. If they lodge an appeal, the LEA must maintain the Statement until the appeal is heard and a decision given, or until the appeal is withdrawn. If parents want to appeal against a decision by the LEA not to maintain their child's Statement, or against changes made to the Statement, they should consult an experienced adviser.

The reform process

When Baroness Warnock published her report in 1978 about inclusion, her heart was in the right place and she was absolutely right to inform the debate about what was happening to our most vulnerable children, who were often being denied an appropriate education and their individual needs were being failed. Baroness Warnock was also correct to want to ensure that Parliament took action through legislation to prevent discriminatory practices in the education system and that society had to protect children with special needs by compelling the local authorities to address the individual needs of the child by ring fencing resources through the means of a Statement.

However, since 2005 she has made it increasingly clear that she has changed her view and feels it is time for a radical review. She has urged government to rethink its framework of inclusion to mean being included in learning, where the child feels they belong rather than just being under the same roof as their peers. She supports the recommendations for reform of the examination system for 14–19-year-olds made in the Tomlinson Review in 2004 but never adopted, and she has urged that there be an independent, apolitical committee of inquiry to make recommendations based on evidence from experts, especially teachers. Although there have been other reports supporting many of her ideas, such as the recommendations made by the House of Commons Education and Skills Committee chaired by Barry Sheerman in 2006 and the Special Educational Consortium under the chairmanship of Brian Lamb which reported in 2009, only a few piecemeal changes have been adopted.

It is now widely accepted that children with special educational needs represent a vast spectrum of need, and society and the education system needs to be diverse and flexible enough to respond to those unique differences.

In March 2011, the UK Government published a Green Paper on special educational needs, with a consultation period to 30 June 2011, which has been dubbed the most radical programme of reforms to hit the area for 30 years. The Green Paper is entitled *Support and Aspiration: A New Approach to Special Educational Needs and Disability* and runs to 120 pages. Here is a summary of these proposals. The goals of the Green Paper include:

- greater integration in the provision of services to children and young people;
- a reduction in bureaucracy and delay;
- greater choice for parents;
- a simpler, less adversarial assessment process free from conflicts of interest.

The most significant proposals are:

- The replacement of Statements and 'statementing' with a single assessment process and a combined education, health and care plan so that health and social services are included in a package of support along with education.
- Such assessments and plans to run from birth up to the age of 25, supporting people through school, further and higher education and into employment.
- The replacement of 'School Action' and 'School Action Plus' with a single 'school based category'. A similar change will be made in relation to Early Years Settings. The aim is to give schools greater flexibility (as well as accountability).
- 'Power to Parents'. This is to be achieved through a number of initiatives including: a requirement that local services publish a 'local offer' showing what support is available and from whom; a legal right, by 2014, for parents to have control of the funds designated for supporting their child; and a greater choice of schools with removal of the bias towards inclusion.
- Involvement of 'the voluntary and community' sector in delivering care plans. Targeted funding will be provided to suitable organizations.
- A reduction in the use of the term 'SEN' and the number of children designated as having special educational needs. This is in accordance with the findings of a report undertaken in 2010 which found that

the term was being overused and large numbers of children wrongly diagnosed.

- Changes to the appeals process, including a right for children to appeal in their own right if they consider they are not getting adequate support. There will also be a greater role for mediation facilitated by an independent party, possibly extending to a requirement that the parties 'always try mediation before an appeal'.

Concluding remarks

It remains to be seen how far the government will take some of the principles and, for example:

- whether control of funding will be passed to all parents on a total and unfettered basis or whether there will be checks and balances;
- what incentives will be given to volunteers, independent organizations, mediators and schools to take up the additional challenges;
- what mechanisms will be put in place to ensure that different bodies act in unison, particularly at a time when they are being encouraged to become independent and pursue their own agendas;
- how the concept of choice can be balanced with the practical considerations of ensuring that specialist services remain viable; and
- how appeals will operate, given the large number of different organizations that will become involved, both in assessing needs and delivering services.

3 Finding support: Practical information for parents and expert witnesses

Statistics relating to the Special Educational Needs and Disability Tribunal (SENDIST)

In 2009–2010, SENDIST mostly heard appeals concerning local authorities' (LAs) refusals to assess a child, or the contents of a Statement or part of it once made. The range of SEN those children had were: autism (26%); specific learning disabilities (dyslexia) (16%); behavioural, social and emotional disabilities (16%); moderate learning disabilities (13%); and speech, language and communication needs (10%). The remainder (19%) comprised physical disabilities, severe learning disabilities, hearing and visual impairments and profound and multiple learning disabilities.

In 2010–2011, a total of 3280 appeals were registered: 17% were legally represented and 7% had a lay representative or parent advocate. Only 22% of appeals lodged led to a full hearing. In 2009–2010, parents were legally represented in 9% of hearings and other parental representatives were present in 11% of cases. LAs were legally represented in 10% of hearings. This indicates that there is settlement in 88% of cases where parents are legally represented, 77% of cases where parents represent themselves (or are withdrawn when parents give up), and only 66% of cases with a support group, charity, lay representative or parent advocate. This is confusing because it puts charities and support groups' free support alongside parent advocate advice which is paid. My experience is that you get what you pay for; some parent advocates are very successful and even amongst specialist education lawyers, some are better than others. It is also true that there is a lot of case law which it is necessary to be aware of; cases do seem to be more complicated and the law can be interpreted in many different ways so that commonsense and the law do not always go together. The conflict is around parents wanting the best for their individual child whereas the LAs only need to provide what is 'adequate' to meet the child's needs. Parents also want to have a fair hearing.

For parents and carers

As stated above, we do not know exactly what the regulations will be for parents to appeal LA decisions following the health, education and social care reforms. However, it is likely that a tribunal system similar to the current one will still be available. Based on the present system, here are matters to consider about the tribunal process.

So you know that your child has some sort of difficulty and is either already in school and not coping, or about to go to school and you are sure that extra help or support will be required. As parents of a child with special needs, one thing is certain: you will need support, advice and information, and it needs to be independent. This is especially important during this period of political, economic and legislative change.

You may be entitled to get Legal Help (or public) funding for financial assistance to fund an education law solicitor who can commission independent expert assessments and reports on your child and help you through whatever the process is for assessment of your child's needs and any appeal process. However, Legal Help will not provide funding for an expert witness to attend a tribunal hearing and may be phased out completely for SEN cases. A specialist solicitor will be able to advise you on whether you are entitled to this. The Law Society (www.lawsociety.org.uk) will be able to give names of solicitors who participate in the Legal Help scheme and are experienced in education law. An exceptional funding scheme is also operated by the Ministry of Justice (MOJ) and Legal Services Commission (LSC), which provides eligible parents with funding for legal representation at hearings where certain criteria are met. Alternatively, you could find support and representation from a support group or charity for free, or enlist a lay representative or parent advocate. Although they charge, their fees are less than a solicitor's. Some useful names and contact details are in the Appendix.

How do you access an independent expert?

You are highly likely to need to find expert witnesses who can assess your child and provide a report and possibly attend the tribunal hearing. You may need advice from your representative as to which of the following are required, and this will of course depend on your child's needs and your case:

- educational psychologist
- speech and language therapist
- occupational therapist
- psychiatrist
- paediatrician
- audiologist
- physiotherapist
- teacher, SENCO or head teacher
- social worker

By 'independent', I mean separate to any of the statutory services. The reason for this is that any professional employed to work in health, education or social services is accountable to their employer and responsible to their line manager. Their job is to provide a service within the constraints of the system and resources and, hopefully, also within the law. They may be individually and personally very lovely people, but they may not tell you about things that their service cannot or are too expensive to provide. In addition, they may not have the time to explore the whole picture with you and listen to and read everyone else's perspective before making conclusions. Of course there are exceptions, and I do not wish to give the impression that on your journey you won't find anyone genuinely caring and helpful employed by health, education or social services. There are shining lights described in some of the personal examples in the following chapters, but I urge you not to take this for granted. Nor do professionals mean to be deliberately unhelpful. Most are doing sterling work against the odds.

Not all professionals working independently will be equally experienced or qualified; however, it is likely that they will have worked at some point for a statutory authority. Some may have made a positive choice to leave completely and set up their own independent practice in order to do things differently, but others will be working part time independently while still working for a statutory authority part time. Like any service you need to purchase, whether double glazing, hairdressing or plumbing, choosing the nearest or the cheapest or the most expensive will not necessarily guarantee best value for money. You need to check out independent professionals in the same way by taking up references, checking professional memberships and insurances and, best of all, by talking to other parents or parent support groups who have been through the process before you. You need to choose the professionals who are going to work with your child extremely carefully. There are certain questions that you should ask and criteria that the professionals need to meet:

- Does the professional have experience in your child's area of special educational need?
- Has the professional been recommended by somebody who has used them for their own child?

You may need a professional to assess your child in order to help you understand their needs fully, or you may need a report to give to the school or the LA for them to understand your child's needs better, or you may need a report in order to appeal to a tribunal. The charities, support groups, lay representatives/parent advocates or solicitors will be able to help you identify professionals, but you will also need to ask the following questions:

- Does the professional have experience of writing reports for tribunals?
- Is the professional able to complete the report within the timeframe and is he/she available to attend the hearing?
- Will the professional attend as an expert witness if requested, and does he/she have experience of tribunals?
- Has the professional attended any expert witness training courses?
- Is the professional a member of the Expert Witness Institute (see Appendix)?

Sometimes, parents ask professionals who are currently working with their child – such as an independent SALT, occupational therapist or dyslexia teacher – to submit a report. This appears to be a good idea as this particular professional should be very knowledgeable about your child's needs and therefore could be deemed to be an 'expert'. However, this does not necessarily mean that their report will be helpful or make them an effective witness if they are not trained to write the type of reports that are required by tribunals. An independent expert professional should know the terminology that is required.

You need to understand that when an independent professional is commissioned to write a report on your child for the purposes of a court hearing or tribunal, you are not paying them to support your child's case. An independent professional expert is exactly what the title says: they are independent and will state their opinion on the child's areas of difficulty and/or need and recommend the provision that, in their professional opinion, they believe is essential for the child to make progress. An independent professional expert's duty is to help the court or tribunal, and if their opinion conflicts with yours, it is of course their duty to say so.

For expert witnesses

Before taking on a case, it is vitally important that professional colleagues consider the following questions:

- Are the special needs of the child iwithin your area of expertise?
- Are you able to produce your report within the necessary timeframe, and are you available to attend as an expert witness if required?
- Do you have time to visit schools? You may be asked to visit to see if the school can deliver the provision that the child needs.
- Do you have a wide range of assessments at your disposal so that you can choose the most relevant one to use?
- If your report is being commissioned by parents, then you must provide them with detailed terms and conditions which clearly outline your fee structure for: reading the background reports; carrying out the assessment; writing the report; and attending the hearing. You also need to make sure that any travel which may be involved is clearly explained so that parents understand what costs might be involved.
- Ask for all the relevant paperwork and reports that have been written on the child, particularly those relating to your profession.
- You will need to liaise with professionals currently working with the child to ensure that assessments are not replicated within too close a timeframe. For example, speech and language therapists cannot usually repeat the same standardized assessment within six months. It is therefore important that contact is made with any treating speech and language therapist in order to determine which assessments have been used. Your professional body may have written guidance on your conduct, writing reports, glossary of terms, communication and liaison.

- It is important that the report is not just about how the child presents in a one-off assessment situation. In most cases, because of the expense involved, parents cannot afford for experts to see their child on several occasions. In order to overcome this, it is essential that the report includes reference to the child's functioning in other environments, such as at home and at school, and, wherever possible, assessments should be carried out in the child's school so that observation can take place. Information can be gained by both parents and teachers. The assessment results should then be compared and contrasted with this information to ensure that they are consistent with the child's general levels of functioning. If they are not, then explanations need to be given. For example, a child with an autistic spectrum condition may do well on standardized language assessments but it is clear from school reports and parent information that they are is struggling to use their language skills appropriately in everyday communicative situations. Therefore, discussion about this needs to form an important part of the report as well as consideration of informal assessments and standardized questionnaires that will elicit the necessary information.
- You need to understand the layout and content for a report for court or tribunal, which must include a preface detailing your areas of experience and expertise.

It is very important that all professionals are aware of the distinction between being an expert in their area of professional knowledge (speech and language therapy, occupational therapy, educational psychology, psychiatry, etc) and being an expert witness. An expert is an individual with experience or knowledge beyond that expected of a typical lay person and who is independently instructed by a court or tribunal to provide evidence. In order to be an expert witness, a professional needs to be qualified both in the content (i.e. their professional knowledge) and the process (of court/tribunals). This is an important distinction, as many professionals make the mistake of thinking that, because they are competent in their job, they are also competent to provide expert evidence. This is not necessarily the case, as an expert witness also needs to be qualified in court processes as well as being an expert in their professional knowledge. This fact has been very clearly illustrated in an article by Jane Ireland (2008). Expert witness courses are available, such as those run by Bond Solon (see Appendix). Expert reports should:

(a) state the purpose for which they were originally written;

(b) set out the substance of all material instructions (whether written or oral) and facts supplied that are relevant to the conclusions and opinions expressed;

(c) give details of any literature or other research material relied on;

(d) describe the assessment process and process of differential diagnosis, highlighting factual assumptions, deductions from those assumptions, and any unusual, contradictory or inconsistent features of the case;

(e) state, with their qualifications, the name of anyone who carried out any test, examination or interview which the expert has used for the report and whether or not that has been carried out under the expert's supervision. State whether other experts have been consulted, at what stage in the process, what information was shared and how this informed the views expressed;

(f) include all relevant information, including confidence in quoted test scores;

(g) identify, narrow and agree any issues where possible;

(h) make it clear if there is not enough information to reach a conclusion on a particular issue, regardless of any pressure to commit to a certainty;

(i) identify any relevant facts not requiring an expert explanation in order to understand or interpret the observation, and description given, as well as any such facts that do require an explanation, e.g. properly conducted examinations or appropriate tests;

(j) highlight any hypotheses or opinions based on peer-reviewed and tested techniques, research and experience accepted as a consensus in the scientific community. Include other relevant background information whether case specific, arising from personal observations, or field specific arising from relevant literature or research;

(k) explain relevant technical subjects, or the meaning and application of applicable technical terms where helpful;

(l) indicate whether an opinion is provisional or qualified, stating the qualification and the reason for it, and identifying what further information is required to give an opinion without qualification;

(m) summarize the range of opinion on any question/issue to be addressed, highlighting and analysing an unknown cause (whether on the facts of the case, e.g. too little information to form a scientific opinion, or due to limited experience, lack of research, peer review or support in the field of their expertise);

(n) summarize opinions expressed with sound reasons for them;

(o) give a clear summary of the recommendations made and clearly date and sign the report.

Reports should also contain the following statement:

I understand that my overriding duty is to assist the tribunal in matters within my expertise, and that this duty overrides any obligation to those instructing me or their clients. I confirm I have complied with that duty and will continue to do so. I confirm that I have made clear which facts and matters referred to in this report are within my own knowledge and which are not. Those that are within my own knowledge I confirm to be true. The opinions I have expressed represent my true and complete opinions on the matters to which they refer.

(Taken from Judge John Aitken, Deputy Chamber President, February 2010)

Concluding remarks

Hopefully, whether you are a parent, carer, lay representative, charity, support group or expert witness, this chapter has given you the background to the current SEN Statementing Process and an indication of what the reforms to the system may be. Whatever the new system, it will remain true that good quality expert evidence may make the difference in your case to SENDIST and pave the way to success for your child's future support, academic and life outcomes.

Part II
Personal Stories

The personal stories that follow have been anonymized. Everyone has given their permission for the stories to be used. However, we appreciate that identity is a fluid thing; people who are happy to share their stories at one point may not like to do so later and therefore anonymity is absolutely vital.

4 Autism and Asperger Syndrome: Communication, friendship and flexibility

Introduction

This chapter features the stories of three children and young people diagnosed with an autistic spectrum condition and the effects these have on their lives, education and families. The stories illustrate different aspects and ages of difficulty and challenge. Arthur's Story is about early intervention, Brandon's Story is about teenage years and Caleb's Story is about entry into adulthood.

Autism

A child with an autistic spectrum condition demonstrates differences in behaviour in all three areas described by Lorna Wing in her triad of impairment (Wing, 1993). These three areas are: verbal communication; social communication; and play, including imagination and flexibility of thought. Sensory hyper/hypo sensitivities also play a huge role in how children with autism are hindered in the learning process. Children with autism learn and succeed in one-to-one structured teaching environments because the steps being taught can be very small and specific. As each skill is learned, the child is then taught how to use the skill in different contexts and settings with lots of repetition and positive reinforcement. Unlike children with other types of conditions, in my experience children with autism need this structured approach to continue beyond the usual school hours and term times if at all possible.

Other children continue to learn naturally from the different experiences they have out of school hours. However, this is often confusing and worrying to children with autism until they have mastered sufficient skills to be able to learn more independently. It is for these reasons that they often make most progress on Applied Behavioural Analysis (ABA) programmes or in specialist ASC school environments.

Autistic spectrum conditions (ASCs) are complex. The educational needs of children with ASCs vary considerably depending on their intellectual ability and their profile of strengths and needs. Staff within all types of school and early education settings where children with an ASC are educated need to understand the implications of ASCs for teaching and learning and should look to modifying the environment and how the curriculum is planned and taught to enable the placement to succeed. As knowledge grows about how children with an ASC think and learn, so the approaches used are constantly modified and developed. Without at least a background knowledge of the challenges that having an ASC can create, a child's behaviour can be misinterpreted and their needs will not be met in the most appropriate way. The emergence of differences in behaviour associated with an ASC in a child places particular stress on the family in addition to the general challenges associated with being a parent.

A whole school approach is the most effective way of meeting the needs of children with an ASC, regardless of type of provision. No matter what type of provision the child is attending, it is important that all staff who might meet the child are aware of the particular needs arising from an ASC. They need to understand the reasons for the child's response to classroom tasks and for their behaviour during lessons and break times.

It is the school's responsibility to ensure that the whole school curriculum is tailored to the needs of children with ASCs. One of the main areas affected by ASCs is understanding the communication of others and communicating effectively with them. Specialists in speech and language are key professionals involved in assessment and intervention.

Early intervention strategies

Some of the interventions not mentioned in the following personal stories that parents have in my experience found helpful for their children are: Early Bird, SPELL, TEACCH, PECS, Intensive Interaction, Musical Interaction Therapy and Applied Behavioural Analysis. They are briefly described below and websites where you can get more information are given in the Appendix.

EarlyBird is a programme designed by the National Autistic Society (NAS) for parents whose child has received a diagnosis of an ASC and is of pre-school age (not yet of statutory school age). The programme aims to support parents in the period between diagnosis and school placement, empowering and helping them facilitate their child's social communication and appropriate behaviour. It helps parents to understand their child's autism: get into their child's world, make contact, and find ways to develop interaction and communication. It also shows also how to analyse and understand the child's behaviours and how to use structure so that problem behaviours can be pre-empted and dealt with. The programme lasts for three months and combines group training sessions with individual home visits, when video feedback is used to help parents apply what they've learned. Parents will have a weekly commitment of a two-and-a-half hour training session or home visit, and to ongoing work with their child at home.

SPELL is an NAS framework for understanding and working with people with an ASC. It stands for structure, positive approaches and expectations, empathy, low arousal and links.

TEACCH (**T**reatment and **E**ducation of **A**utistic and **C**ommunication related handicapped **CH**ildren) is an evidence-based service, training and research programme for individuals of all ages and skill levels with ASCs developed in North Carolina in the 1970s.

The Picture Exchange Communication System (PECS) is a successful approach that uses pictures or symbols to develop communication skills. It is appropriate for children and adults with learning and communication difficulties including autism.

Intensive interaction is an approach to teaching the pre-speech fundamentals of communication to children and adults who have severe learning difficulties and/or autism and who are still at an early stage of communication development.

Musical Interaction Therapy was developed by Wendy Prevezer, SALT at Sutherland House School in Nottingham, specifically for developing communication skills in children with ASC. It is currently being evaluated scientifically by Dr Dawn Wimpory at Bangor University.

Applied Behavioural Analysis (ABA)

ABA programmes for children with autism are based on an analysis of what motivates an individual child and each skill the child needs to learn is broken down into small, achievable steps. Each step is worked on in a systematic and consistent way, using appropriate reinforcement to encourage the behaviours needed. Evidence and data are collected of the child's progress, so that targets and motivators can be adjusted along the way according to what is and isn't working for the particular child. Reinforcement systems – which seek to link desired behaviour with good outcomes or rewards for the child – are particularly important for children with autism, given they may lack the 'social desire to please' that is often present in a normally-functioning child. ABA teaches a child how to learn, and can therefore be applied to the widest range of skills – from speech and language, self-care and motor skills, right through to reading and writing.

Results from a meta analysis of early behavioural intervention for children with autism by Eldevik et al. (2009) support the clinical implication that at present, and in the absence of other interventions with established efficacy, early intensive behavioural intervention (ABA) should be an intervention of choice for children with autism.

Hayward et al. (2009) published a ground-breaking study in ABA as it is one of the few outcome studies to have been conducted in the UK. Findings are consistent with previous studies demonstrating the effectiveness of ABA treatment for children with autism.

ABA has a rich scientific history in assisting those with developmental disabilities and there is a vast body of research, spanning four decades, documenting its effectiveness for children with autism. Indeed, a number of systematic reviews of evidence-based practices in autism conclude that ABA input in the early years for children with autism has the strongest evidence base of any comprehensive intervention (Eldevik et al, 2009; Rogers, 2008).

ABA is also called Early Intensive Behavioural Intervention (EIBI) or Intensive Behavioural Intervention (IBI). Verbal Behaviour (VB) is a branch of ABA which focuses more on teaching in the natural environment through experiences. Any professional leading a home ABA programme needs to be a Board Certified Behaviour Analyst (BCBA). A BCBA will work in collaboration with other professionals, sharing resources and keeping the child's best interest at the forefront.

Arthur's story

This could be a very long story, but to cut it extremely short: Arthur is the younger of our two sons and (after a bit of a battle with what appeared to be everyone at that time) was diagnosed with autism (at the more severe end of the spectrum) at the tender age of 22 months! Following lots of appointments with various different professionals (with all the associated negativity), we were getting no further forward with making sense of anything. Arthur was spiralling out of control and it seemed as though there was absolutely nothing that we could do!

In sheer desperation, I found an independent speech and language therapist's (SALT)number in an NAS publication and made contact to see if there was any way she could help us. Our initial appointment consisted of an interview in the therapist's home. Thereafter, Arthur and I visited weekly over quite a substantial period of time. The SALT devised a list'of 10 or so items/activities each week that we were to work on. Obviously, initially there were only one or two things that were appropriate. Using these 'positives' we worked forwards with a programme that, once we had completed a few weeks, Arthur and I could successfully complete most of the items on an A4 sheet. With all this success we became much more motivated than we had been in the previous months.

As the weeks went on, the SALT put us in touch with all sorts of other therapists that could support us. Arthur had problems with sleep (he basically never slept through the night, and once up would 'play'). We were introduced to a sound therapist, who devised a tape for Arthur to listen to before he went to bed. This worked wonders! He wore headphones (we never thought he would); and sat spellbound with this 'music' for about an hour before he went to bed. This was reviewed and he still uses a very similar therapy to this day.

Arthur has always been very 'hyper' and 'bouncy'! Although there is nothing really wrong with this, there are obviously times when this isn't always appropriate. Time to call in a nutritional therapist. She recognized that there were certain foods that would spark off this unconventional behaviour. With lots of support and guidance, we adopted a casein- and gluten-free diet. Although we relaxed this just a couple of years ago, we still recognize certain rules, especially when out and about and on holidays.

Once a child with special needs goes to school, they need to have a Statement (or at least have one in progress). Without the SALT's guidance (as with everything else, I didn't have the first clue), and an introduction to a specialist special educational needs solicitor, Arthur most certainly wouldn't have benefited from all the support, love and specialized care of the residential ASC specific school he attends today following a successful appeal to SENDIST.

I have kept a diary. Although it makes me cry buckets, it is sometimes worth an hour or so to look them out and remind myself of what we have as a family coped with and have successfully come through. More importantly, we take time to celebrate all the achievements that Arthur makes every day, no matter how small they may appear to others. For us now, everything is extremely special, and time spent together as a family is important.

There were times when we were just so wrapped up in the 'negatives' that it was impossible to see anything positive. It was extremely upsetting that Arthur did not talk, wouldn't want to associate with anyone, wrapped himself in his own little world and wouldn't let anyone in. The SALT would always be there to support and was always insistent that this was just a 'phase' that he was going through. I most certainly didn't believe her at the time, but we are now on a totally different chapter. His speech is not as good as it could be; but it gets him what he needs! He is always curious about new people; and always has a cuddle when he has missed us.

This is just a very brief synopsis of all the hard work that has gone on over the past ten years. Every chapter brings in new challenges, with new goal posts that are ever needing to be moved.

We never say never these days. As a family we spend many a happy hour together. Arthur has a love of socialising and loves a restaurant and good food. He loves days out 'and is always beautifully behaved. We even go abroad for our holidays these days!

Asperger syndrome

In a draft released in February 2010, the American Psychiatric Association's DSM – V (*Diagnostic and Statistical Manual of Mental Disorders, Fifth Edition*) has proposed to eliminate the diagnosis of Asperger Syndrome and instead group it together with autism. However, it is included as a separate diagnosis in this book. People diagnosed with Asperger Syndrome (AS) do not show early language delay and will be of at least average intelligence. Verbal delay is not necessarily seen in AS but there is a substantial degree of disordered language development, very frequently shown partly in echolalia, but invariably shown in semantic/pragmatic disorder. Insofar as AS is a coding disorder (a difficulty with making sense of certain areas of experience), there is a relationship between ASC/AS and dyslexia where the difficulty is focused on reading and writing. It is not unusual to find AS and dyslexia associated in the same person.

It is usual for children with AS to show spontaneous improvement but this tends to be surface level and the child remains fragile and in need of massive support if the improvement is to be maintained. Further improvement is to be expected into adulthood. Depressive breakdown is quite common in adolescence and early adulthood and is often reactive to loss of self-esteem where the complexities of AS have not been adequately recognized or as a reaction to bullying. The triad of impairments dating from before 3 years of age applies to the child with AS as to the less able child with autism as follows.

Developmental impairment of language of a semantic/pragmatic nature. Common in AS is where a child doesn't understand meaning because he fails to empathize with the intention of the speaker or where he doesn't understand the significance in context of what he himself has said as a result of a lack of empathy. The pragmatics of language refers to the in-built skills which make language communicative and usable in practice. These include: gesture and facial expression; social timing (to achieve flow of spoken language between people); listening skills, including body language, that convey attention and picking up other people's body language; appropriate distance and volume; intonation; eye contact; and so on.

Social impairment, especially social empathy. Many children with AS learn to respond to social ambiguities on paper but cannot generalize this to situations.

Rigidity and inflexibility of thinking and behaviour. This shows itself in various ways according to the child's age and ability and includes verbal behaviour. Common aspects are: repetitive play; lack of pretend play; preference for patterns; repetitive speech including echoing; fixed, repetitive interests; pedantic speech; difficulty with generalization and adaptation.

The following recommendations are informed by current knowledge of pupils with AS and how they manage in mainstream school:

- many people with AS are capable of acquiring normal academic qualifications;
- many people with AS become clinically depressed in adolescence and adulthood. This is more likely if they are unemployed, thus it is especially helpful for a person with AS to acquire qualifications which will have value in the employment market.

Depression is often the result of:

- insufficient attention to the emotional aspects of a person lacking social skills and finding himself shunned;

- active teasing, and often bullying, which tends to increase if not attended to pro-actively. On the whole a smaller school is preferable.

Pupils with AS need direct support and teaching from specialist teachers who are skilled and experienced in working with pupils with autistic spectrum conditions. These teachers should have on-going professional development to inform them of the most appropriate means of supporting those with autism as reflected in both research and practice. Ideally, such a specialist teacher will have completed a distance learning course in autism, such as the ones run at Birmingham University, University of Wales, Newport, Bangor University or Sheffield Hallam University. Pupils may also need the following:

- an individual timetable focusing on organizational elements of a task;
- use of an individual workstation to minimize distractibility and promote independence on task behaviour for specified activities.

These types of approaches would not need to be applied intensively and the degree of implementation could usefully be judged and modified with access to specialist staff. Pupils with AS need to be closely monitored so they don't get lost in the system.

Pupils with AS also needs a structured programme designed to help them overcome some of their planning and organizational difficulties and a structured programme of activities to develop their social and communication skills. Areas to focus on include direct teaching of:

- learning to appreciate and understand the needs of a listener;
- teaching reciprocal conversational skills with a focus on rules of conversation;
- working on topic maintenance skills and self-monitoring of language use;
- identifying how much spoken detail is appropriate to different social contexts;
- continuing to teach more ambiguous language terms in very direct ways;
- direct teaching of emotions and interpretation/appropriate use of nonverbal gestures;
- prediction of likely outcomes in social events/contexts.

The achievement of pro-social goals by children and the consequent acceptance by peers and leaders build self-confidence and esteem, encouraging further skills development. The role of peers in social skills training is seen as critical. Peers act as adjunct trainers, modelling skills, sharing reinforcement contingencies and providing mutual feedback, which supports the acquisition and maintenance of new social skills and attitudes attainable through awareness training of pupils and teaching staff. Teachers can only promote peer trainers if they themselves have positive attitudes towards children with special needs. Tolerance and understanding need to be actively taught.

The specific aims of social skills programmes are to develop:

- social perception, particularly listening to and looking carefully at others to recognize individual differences and similarities and to take the perspective of others;
- communication skills, particularly recognizing, naming and expressing feelings appropriately;
- verbal and non-verbal behavioural skills, including friendly approach behaviours, conversational, self-protective and assertive skills;
- cognitive problem-solving skills, particularly defining social problems and personal goals, generating solutions, evaluating consequences, making decisions and initiating actions;
- democratic conflict resolution skills requiring mutual respect, shared responsibility and self-control;
- awareness of socially acceptable or morally responsible strategies for resolving social conflicts;
- techniques for maintaining friendships;
- group membership skills, including active participation, cooperation, leadership and democratic group decision-making and problem-solving skills.

A pupil with AS would find it difficult to access the curriculum without developing these communication and social skills and that is why I consider that it is appropriate for a specialist speech and language therapist to develop these skills as an educational provision. With early intensive intervention, a wide variety of behaviours associated with social skills impairment such as school phobia, depression, conduct disorders, poor self-esteem and bullying may be avoided.

Brandon's story

Brandon's parents themselves negotiated the wording of his SEN Statement with their local education authority, which included specified and quantified provision for him to have social skills group therapy in primary school and in the holidays over a period of about five years. Brandon's parents also attended a 'Stop, Think, Do' (Petersen and Lewis, 2004) parents group. It is their belief that this combination of integrated and consistent therapy, with parents, therapists and education staff working together, helped to achieve the following results.

Brandon has just gone from strength to strength. He finished secondary school in the summer with three 'A' passes at 'A' level. He represented the local Rotary Club at a conference in Europe last year and came back to give a Powerpoint presentation at a Rotary Club dinner.

He won the Student of the Year award in Year 12 and in his last year won the school's prize for outstanding achievement and originality. He has grown into a remarkable young man of whom we are very proud. He has established a great group of friends from school with whom he keeps in touch on MSN and Facebook. He has now gone to university and so far seems to have settled into the social life. We are not sure if he is doing any work!

Caleb's story

Caleb was the second child to be diagnosed to be autistic in a small unitary local authority when he was 3 years old. This meant there was very little understanding of how it affected him and, as a family, we had no professional support or advice in relation to how to help him or how to manage his behaviour for many years. Caleb was placed in a language unit attached to a primary school in another area – some distance from where we live. Although he received SALT and had additional support in class, there was no understanding of how his autism affected him. He did not learn to read until he was 10 years old – and had to be taught using Rebus Symbols. He then had to be re-taught to read at home, because he could not transfer his learning into a different environment. Caleb continues to struggle with generalizing his learning and he cannot multi-task.

Caleb had full-time support as he simply could not process information. Unfortunately, this made him the target of school bullies. It started in primary school when a gang of bullies pushed him in the urinal. After this, he never used the toilet at school again.

He became a highly vulnerable teenager. At high school, he was introduced to smoking and he then went on to become addicted to both alcohol and drugs. His extremely high social vulnerability continues to affect him on a daily basis. He cannot recognize when people are using him.

When Caleb left school at 19 years old, he made it clear that he wanted to work and we encouraged him in this as we felt it would be good for his self-esteem. After having had a support assistant at school, for which he was bullied, he resisted the idea of having a support worker in a work situation. The Careers Adviser at high school had told Caleb that if he went into catering he would never be out of work. However, the Adviser had no idea how Caleb's autism made it very difficult for him to process information quickly, to be able to multi-task, plan or deal with changes in rotas, numbers, etc. Nor was the Careers Adviser aware of Caleb's health difficulties (e.g. recognizing and identifying internal pain) or his sleep disorder. All of this made catering very difficult for Caleb.

Caleb lacks the ability to understand/be aware of internal pain – if he cannot see it then it does not exist, until it has become so very bad that it is beyond belief (tooth abscesses, severe tonsillitis, ear infections) which is dangerous because he does not show the usual reaction to pain. We have been advised that a small percentage of people with ASC have this feature and it is called a 'neglect of pain'.

Because Caleb stopped using the toilet at school, he went all day (from when he left at 7.30am till he got home again at 4pm) without using the toilet. With most people, the pain would force them to go. Eventually, his tubes seized up and he was rushed to hospital. It took four operations to widen the tubes. He still gets the pain – and still needs to self-catheterize. However, he is still unaware of the pain until it has reached an extreme level. Caleb has, we have been told, an 'oppositional' reaction to medications, that is, he has adverse reactions to most medications that help most people. For example, medication for depression made him feel invincible.

We tried to help Caleb with his independence by creating a 'chill out' shed at the end of the garden, which is adjacent to a back entrance. Sadly, people he thought were his friends took advantage – one night, two introduced him to a new way of smoking cannabis (which involved chest compressions). Unknown to us, Caleb lost consciousness and hit his head on the concrete. He became quite noticeably autistic – repeating the same phrase over and over again. It took a very long time for Caleb to recover from this – and his memory has been affected.

Caleb finds it really difficult to do any of the kind of daily planning that most people take for granted. For example, he has never had any idea of planning his day – having the right things with him for what he wants to do, budgeting, having lunch, etc. He has no idea when his clothes are dirty or when his bedding needs changing. He finds it impossible to deal with forms as he cannot understand what the questions mean. He cannot take phone messages – and cannot cope with telephone calls unless he knows the people calling him. He cannot, as yet, use email. His use of computers is only about researching cars, which is his area of special interest.

Caleb has real problems with sleeping – this has been since he was a baby. Melatonin helps (without it he does not sleep at all) and he was the first person in the area to be prescribed Melatonin for problems with sleeping associated with ASC. But some nights he still can't sleep, usually because he's anxious about something or because it's a sign that he's unwell.

Caleb also does not seem to understand the need to eat regularly. When he's busy he just does not stop – and his low blood sugar then makes him very irritable. But he does not learn from this so it just goes on and on. We've tried to encourage him to eat regularly, reminding him, and trying to ensure he's got enough money to buy himself lunch.

Our local authority was one of the pilot areas for Personal Budgets and Caleb was one of the first to be awarded a Personal Budget. His Care Manager had advised us that Caleb really needed a 24-hour residential placement but was aware that there was nowhere appropriate for him locally. So we worked out a Support Plan that would enable him to develop his learning. With the agreement of his Care Manager we found and helped Caleb to rent a little lockup garage on a small industrial estate. Several of the people (older than Caleb) running motor maintenance businesses have been very supportive to Caleb and they seem genuinely concerned about him.

Caleb now has somewhere of his own, which has helped his self-esteem. BUT he thought he could do the car maintenance on his own. He found, of course, that he could not. In the end, his dad has had to help him as he has always had an interest in cars and had previously been a support worker on the Motor Maintenance course at the college. Caleb completed his Level 1 course at the local college. We had to do all the paperwork for him and the Learning Support department at our request arranged online access to a specialist resource – but again he needs his dad's support to be able to understand and access this.

This year, his dad signed up to do a Level 2 with Caleb. They have both just passed their Level 2 with Distinction. His dad was able to prompt Caleb – to check he remembered his safety equipment and folders. He kept Caleb going when the demands increased. No one knew that his dad was supporting him which meant Caleb's self-esteem was maintained.

Now the challenges continue as Caleb and his dad are going to try to develop the lockup into a commercial enterprise. It is likely to take a long time but we hope that, by enabling Caleb to learn the skills he needs, doing an activity he finds motivating and enjoys, he will continue to make progress. He will need a high level of support to turn his lockup, which has functioned as a training workshop, into a business. He's going to have to learn to understand paperwork. One of the biggest challenges is going to be to remember to charge his mobile phone!

But we believe in him. What we try to encourage is for Caleb to start believing in himself.

Concluding remarks

What works for young people with ASC or AS will vary depending on their personality, cognitive ability, the severity of their autism and degree of learning disability. But it is clear from Arthur, Brandon and Caleb's stories that support, information and training for the family from diagnosis onwards is essential, alongside accurate assessment of needs, a range of therapies and interventions, and placement in an appropriate school which may be a local mainstream school or a specialist ASC provision. Speech and language therapy to work on both communication and social, relationship and friendship skills, and occupational therapy for both motor skills and sensory issues, are essential in any provision alongside an appropriate behaviour management programme.

The role of ICT, nutrition and physical activity are often integrated into a specialist curriculum in order to progress independence and life skills. And these support services need to continue into adulthood for many.

5 Behavioural, emotional and social conditions: Learning, feelings and mood

Introduction

Behavioural, emotional and social conditions describe a range of symptoms such as depression, anxiety, fears and phobias. The following chapter includes the personal stories of Dexter and Ernest who both have a diagnosis of Attention Deficit Hyperactivity Disorder. (ADHD) Dexter is now an adult and his story describes the support that helped him and his family on their journey. Ernest is still at primary school but has other competing factors which make his support needs more complex.

Attention Deficit Hyperactivity Disorder

One of the most common conditions to affect learning is Attention Deficit Hyperactivity Disorder (ADHD). Children with ADHD are sometimes inattentive, hyperactive and impulsive. They can have a short attention span, be restless, easily distracted, and constantly fidget. They may take regular medication to help control these behaviours. In the UK, about 1.7% of the population, mostly children, have ADD or ADHD. Boys are more likely to be affected. A child with ADD or ADHD might show the following symptoms.

Attention difficulties

- does not pay close attention to detail or makes careless errors during work or play;
- does not finish tasks or sustain attention in play activities;
- seems not to listen to what is said to him or her;

- does not follow through instructions or finish homework or chores (not because of confrontational behaviour or failure to understand instructions);
- is disorganized about tasks and activities;
- avoids tasks like homework that require sustained mental effort;
- loses things necessary for certain tasks or activities, such as pencils, books or toys;
- is easily distracted;
- is forgetful in the course of daily activities.

Hyperactivity

- runs around or excessively climbs over things (in adolescents or adults, only feelings of restlessness may occur);
- unduly noisy in playing, or has difficulty in engaging in quiet leisure activities;
- leaves seat in classroom or in other situations where remaining seated is expected;
- fidgets with hands or feet or squirms on seat.

Impulsivity

- blurts out answers before the questions have been completed;
- does not wait in line or await turns in games or group situations;
- interrupts or intrudes on others, e.g. butts into others' conversations or games;
- talks excessively without appropriate response to social restraint;
- is destructive, such as tearing pages out of books or breaking equipment, even if remorseful afterwards.

The young person with this diagnosis will show the above difficulties in all settings, e.g. at school/college and at home.

Dexter's story

Dexter was on the go all the time from his first steps at the age of 15 months. He was into everything and did not sleep properly through the night until he was nearly 5. He was not able to sit down and focus on drawing or inset puzzles at nursery, and preferred to be up running around and flitting from activity to activity. Dexter's parents were exhausted and found that their extended family were not keen to look after him as he would not occupy himself but rather needed continual adult attention to get him to focus.

By the start of primary school, Dexter had fractured his clavicle and elbow from jumping off trees and from heights. He was often in the casualty department and his parents joked that he had a season ticket to attend there.

During infant school, Dexter struggled to sit still at circle time and was not popular with his peers. Parents of other children complained about him to the school and to other parents in the playground. The school SENCO discussed the class teacher's concerns with the parents. Dexter was referred by the GP to the local community paediatrics team who recommended parent training around positive reinforcement, and also giving him some additional support to remain on task in school at School Action Plus of the Code of Practice.

His parents read *1-2-3 Magic* and joined a parenting group. They were relieved that something was being done and that they were not being blamed as bad parents. After all, they had two older boys with no difficulties at all.

After a six-month trial of positive behavioural management and parenting classes, the parents were less punitive and found that there had been a short-term response to praise and clear targets. They had also given Dexter omega-3 fish oils for three months but with no improvement. However, the progress did not last, and he continued to 'be all over the place'. He was not able to sit and watch a film all the way through without getting up and making a nuisance of himself. He could not sit at the table for meals and he had no friends at school. His morale was low and he was struggling to read.

The community paediatrician discussed medication options with the parents, who initially were sceptical as they were worried about side effects of using medication with such a young child (Dexter was now aged 7). However, on reflection and after careful reassurance, they decided that something needed to improve, as Dexter was being excluded for disruptive behaviour and hitting his peers. He seemed to be gravitating towards all the 'problem children' at the school.

Dexter's parents agreed to undertake a trial of stimulant medication, mainly to address Dexter's school day, as they thought they could manage him after school by giving him more one-to-one attention. Initially, Dexter complained of some stomach pains and loss of appetite, but this passed after a few days. As the dose was increased to match his weight, Dexter's restlessness, impulsiveness and inattention improved. He started to read for the first time and began to try homework. After a few months, he was being invited to parties for the very first time; his parents were in tears of joy as they had been so worried about his social isolation.

The primary school took advice from the behaviour support specialist teacher service and instigated individualized approaches with as much one-to-one time with his teaching assistant as possible. Increased computer-based learning helped his focus; egg timers were employed to help with time management and awareness. Dexter was provided with a 'tangle', a plastic spiral which allowed him to fiddle with his hands under the table and not distract other children near him. He sat on a table close to the teacher so that he did not have the additional distraction of people in front of him. Tactical ignoring of attention-seeking behaviour and use of visual cards to prompt him to remain on task were found to work. Target charts were used between home and school to reward him for clear goals and immediate rewards were given wherever possible. Dexter was placed with good role models to help him with learning appropriate behaviour. Nuisance items such as rubber bands and rulers were strategically removed, whilst activity reinforcement was employed using the less desirable task before the more desirable reward task. His parents were included as partners in Dexter's success. Close home–school liaison was maintained by email and diaries, with the focus on the positives and reinforcing targets.

Exercise was found to promote Dexter's focus. He enjoyed football and could concentrate better in a team, although he needed prompting when group instructions were given. The parents joined ADDIS UK and the local ADHD support network for parents.

Careful planning for the transition to secondary school was undertaken, involving both SENCOs and the community paediatrician. Dexter's parents had worked hard to identify a school which had a sympathetic ethos and an understanding of the need for supporting children with poor organizational skills, differentiation of class work, homework and after-school clubs. They found a school which also provided nurturing for the Year 7 transition and had good links with the local community paediatric and CAMHS teams.

Dexter's medication needed to be changed to a preparation which covered the early evenings as well as the school day and a suitable longer-acting preparation of Methylphenidate was started. Dexter's sleep pattern needed help as his medication kept him awake, so he took Melatonin to help his sleep pattern at night, which worked.

Although Dexter struggled with organizational issues, and low level disruption, the school implemented a Pastoral Support Plan and also involved educational psychology and specialist teaching advice to keep him from being excluded. He was helped by having structured activities during his breaks and also found swimming in the local club helped him to burn off energy.

However, he struggled in Year 9 with secondary challenging behaviour and cannabis misuse, and ran into several fixed-term exclusions. After a period of time in a local pupil referral unit, his parents requested a statutory assessment. The LA refused and continued to believe that Dexter could manage within mainstream education. Dexter's parents appealed to the SEND Tribunal and used a strong letter of support from the consultant child psychiatrist and ADHD nurse. The parents requested a representative from an SEN charity to support them at the appeal. The LA backed down and agreed to assess Dexter the day before the tribunal. The local authority issued a Statement of Special Educational Needs but found that the local BESD school was full.

Dexter was managed within an alternative curriculum involving small group tuition in the home of a tutor from an independent organization. He responded very well to this and also was transferred to CAMHS due to the possibility of substance-related psychosis from the cannabis.

Dexter commenced Risperidone alongside his long-acting stimulant and he settled down with additional substance misuse counselling. Dexter managed to gain enough GCSEs to attend a local college where he was able to take up a practical-based NVQ course around carpentry. At the age of 18, the local CAMHS team found it hard to get his care managed by local adult mental health services so he was referred to the South London and Maudsley Adult ADHD service whereby his GP was happy to continue prescribing under their advice.

Dexter continued with his apprenticeship in carpentry, living at home with his parents, and managed to gain a job locally with a building firm. He found that by his early 20s he no longer needed medication to focus as he was much more in charge of his working day and activities rarely required him to focus in a group. He settled down with a steady girlfriend who was a good organizer and helped him with time management, and eventually moved in with her.

Ernest's story

In contrast with the above, Ernest's story is still ongoing and his diagnosis has been complicated by his early life experiences and the attachment disorder which is common to many Looked After Children (fostered and adopted children). He also has a severe medical condition which makes treatment and management less straightforward. Ernest's story is told by his Special Guardians.

Ernest was born with a rare but severe and life-threatening heart abnormality, diagnosed by scan before birth. His birth mother was very young and unable to provide the necessary care for his significant health and care needs. Ernest's medical condition is not curable. All treatment is palliative. The best guess is that he will need a heart transplant when he is a teenager. Ernest was initially not expected to survive; however, given his progress there is now a 97% chance of him surviving into adulthood.

Ernest had his first open heart surgery at 3 days old, his second stage open heart surgery at 3 months old, and was placed in a secure placement away from home aged just 4 months on discharge from hospital because there were no trained foster carers where he lived who could cope with a naso-gastric tube. During his period in care he had many different carers, often on a 24-hour shift basis followed by three days off. As a result of this experience, Ernest has developed an attachment disorder.

Ernest was tube fed for five months and was developmentally delayed. He didn't walk unaided until he was 19 months old. Before that, he bottom shuffled rather than crawled. He had physiotherapy, OT, speech and language therapy, play therapy, hydrotherapy and was known to the educational psychologist. We immediately offered our family as either a long-term kinship foster or adoptive placement for Ernest. We are a professional couple with three birth children of our own, a large house and support systems already in place. Ernest was placed with us when he was 21 months old. When he arrived, he only had about 20 single words he could say clearly.

Ernest attended nursery when he was 2.5 years old. He started with two mornings a week, increasing to five mornings a week aged 3 years. From age 3.5 years, Ernest attended a nursery class every morning. He was able to cope much more normally in an environment with small classes and a high level of adults to children. His attention needed constant refocusing and he was therefore better able to cope in a structured environment where he was directed and knew what was expected of him at all times. He was worried by a lot of coming and going and changes of personnel. When anxious, he would try to escape, so the physical environment needed to be safe and secure. His behaviour and noise level escalated if he felt in need of reassurance or attention. He would copy the behaviour of children whom he perceived as getting more attention than him.

For his emotional development we were advised that Ernest needed to learn how to both monitor and modify his own behaviour and having a 1:1 TA would not be at all helpful to him. There were no concerns about his hearing or vision. His speech and language skills were age appropriate. Ernest is and is likely to remain on the physically small side for his chronological age. He is seen regularly by a dentist and needs to brush his teeth three times a day after meals to minimize the risk of endocarditis. He needs a high calorie diet and encouragement to eat enough little and often and to drink cold fluids in summer and warm fluids in winter. He can join in physical activity appropriate to his age but is not able to do contact sport due to his chest scar. He needs supervision at playtimes. He tires easily, especially in extremes of weather. Ernest needs to be under the supervision of a responsible adult at all times as he has difficulties with balance, fine motor coordination (manipulation) and concentration. Ernest is seen regularly by a GP regarding his development and medication. Emotionally, Ernest doesn't completely trust anybody although he appears smiley and happy on the surface. He is demanding, overfriendly and attention seeking, particularly with strangers. He is often inconsiderate of others' feelings and will deliberately damage toys or models, for example.

Ernest is often defiant, disobedient and disruptive at home and school. He finds it hard to make friends and mix with other children. He rushes into everything without thinking and finds it difficult to settle to any task for more than a few moments. He will 'steal' toys from his brothers' bedrooms without asking and can be destructive. He is restless and fidgety. He will overeat if allowed to. He equates food with care and if denied food he becomes very distressed because he thinks he is not loved.

Despite his average cognitive and developmental skills, Ernest has a combination of difficulties which result in him having recognized needs in the areas of health, education, identity, family and social relationships, emotional and behavioural development and self-care skills. It is for these reasons that we requested a statutory assessment of his special educational needs, delayed school placement and then placement in a small, structured, caring school with small classes in a safe, secure and supportive environment where he can lead as normal and happy a life for as long as possible. If possible, we wanted all three of our primary school-aged children to be in the same school. This was partly so that we did not have to be in two places at once at the beginning and end of the school day but also for Ernest's security, both for attachment reasons and safety at playtime.

On the advice of our solicitors, we commissioned expert reports from a consultant psychiatrist and an independent occupational therapist. They described in detail each and every one of his special educational needs so that we had a much better understanding of what Ernest needed to progress. Ernest was diagnosed with an emerging ADHD presentation and sensory issues which were not just related to his medical condition but also to his disorganized thought processes as a result of his early experiences.

The SENDIST hearing was set for when Ernest was exactly 4.5 years of age and the witnesses were to have been an independent educational psychologist and the NHS specialist clinical psychologist for fostering and adoption. We were represented by a leading education law barrister. Later, the LEA stated that they agreed the school placement on the basis of Ernest's attachment disorder. Ernest could *not* have managed in the local primary school, regardless of the support provided, because of the complexity of his needs and the head teacher of that school told our EP that she thought he should go to a school for children with severe learning difficulties. If this is the basis of the LEA's decision, they never communicated it with us or any of our solicitors. However, the LEA did see the bigger picture and did communicate with our solicitors and in fact negotiated without the need for a SENDIST hearing.

Four years later, Ernest is attending a local state-maintained primary school but they are struggling to implement his Statement in a holistic and integrated way. He has full-time TA support but he regards them as his personal slaves and often refuses to do any work. He is therefore close to the bottom of his class although he is of average cognitive ability with above average language. He has therefore recently undergone a Statutory Reassessment. Our independent educational psychologist has diagnosed dyslexia and the consultant child and adolescent psychiatrist has confirmed that he has a marked attachment disorder of an insecure and disinhibited nature, very high anxiety and fluctuating attention (emergent ADHD), Oppositional Defiant Disorder, poor balance and coordination and is at a high risk of developing antisocial behavioural problems. Ernest needs an intensive behavioural programme and intensive psychotherapy as an educational need.

The initial reaction of the LA was to issue a proposed amended Statement which is vague and hard to read and has not quantified or specified provision, completely ignoring the expert medical and psychological advice. We have once again instructed a solicitor to negotiate with the LA and appeal the Statement if necessary. It would seem that even with our background and knowledge, excellent support and a good, caring local authority we still have to fight every step of the way to get the support that this child needs to have as normal a life as possible.

Concluding remarks

It is important to remember when living and working with children with challenging behaviour that many children are incorrectly diagnosed due to an undetected acquired brain injury. This chapter leaves no doubt about the complexity of both the special educational needs of a child with a social, emotional or behavioural condition, and the fight that parents/guardians may have to take on in order to get the support required for a positive future for their child. It should be remembered that not all parents may have the capacity or capability to undertake this challenge, and it is up to professionals to work towards this positive future for the child on their behalf. It is also true that children who have language and communication difficulties are likely to have some learning processes disrupted such as attention, organizing and retrieving information, generalizing learning from one context to another, speed of learning and ability to assimilate experience. Whilst children may see and hear things around them it does not always follow that they will pay attention or listen. Attention and listening are selective. They are processes which the child gradually comes to control consciously. The ability to focus attention and to ignore distractions involves higher order processes.

In my experience, there is a strong link between language ability and behaviour. Popularity among peers is affected by the child's intelligence, friendliness, physical attractiveness and physical size. Aggression among children seems initially to be a response to frustration. The form and amount of aggression changes with age. Associations between language problems and behaviour problems have been extensively documented. It is held that frustration experienced by children with language needs, because they cannot communicate effectively, leads to acting out behaviour. Language provides a framework for thinking which may be used to regulate arousal and emotional states. Children with ADHD are considered to be at greater risk of having SLCN and later of having higher rates of anxiety disorders, aggressive behaviour and increased substance abuse. Developing support services for young people with behavioural, emotional and social conditions, with or without additional speech language and communication needs, is vital if we as a society are to support young people to achieve their potential and not slide into offending or have secondary mental health needs including addictions. Dexter has achieved this and we hope Ernest will, too.

6 Specific learning disability, dyslexia and dyscalculia: Reading, writing and calculating

Introduction

Some individuals with dyslexia may also have spoken language needs, although some may not, so I make no apology for the fact that the three personal stories presented here are children and young people who have both written and spoken language needs. This chapter contains the personal stories of Fatima, Gabriel and Harvey. All have been supported in specialist schools or colleges for pupils with severe dyslexia which also have speech and language therapy and occupational therapy as integral to the teaching. Fatima did not get this specialist support until she was 15 but Gabriel and Harvey transferred to a specialist school in their primary school years. All had received good support from either speech and language therapists or teachers but their needs required more specialist and integrated intervention to enable them to make progress.

Dyslexia

The Rose Report (2009) describes dyslexia as a 'learning difficulty that primarily affects the skills involved in accurate and fluent word reading and spelling… A good indication of the severity and persistence of dyslexic type difficulties can be gained by examining how the individual has responded to well founded intervention'.

Children may therefore be considered to have dyslexia if, in spite of adequate teaching, they have specific persistent needs with reading and writing in comparison with their abilities in other spheres to a degree sufficient to prevent school work reflecting their true ability and knowledge Early identification of dyslexia is essential if these children are to receive appropriate support. The earlier the needs are identified, the greater the likelihood of success. The personal story of a child with dyslexia may reveal early, previously undiagnosed language needs that only become of recognized significance in the light of emerging reading and writing needs.

A full multidisciplinary assessment of a child with severe dyslexia should include an educational psychologist, occupational therapist, teacher, audiologist, orthoptist and paediatrician in addition to a speech and language therapist.

In therapy given for dyslexia, the therapist must be aware of the relationship between spoken and written language needs. As deficits in phonological awareness and processing are often key features of dyslexia, speech and language therapists' knowledge and skills and their training in phonetics mean that they are ideally placed to contribute to the management of children with dyslexia. Informed phonetics and linguistic techniques have proven to be successful. In addition, when providing therapy to children with spoken language needs, the SALT will consider prerequisite written language skills and actual written language skills as part of the overall intervention programme. The discharge of a child who is speaking but not reading or writing or showing prerequisite skills appropriate to age cannot be seen as a successful discharge. Intervention will be offered that utilizes the skills of teaching staff at all times.

When planning intervention, teachers and therapists will be aware of the emotional reaction that the existence of reading and writing needs provokes in both the child and carer. Frustration and evasion are understandable sequallae to the educational problems and daily ordeal of school work for these children. Children who have good speech and language skills are at an advantage when they learn to read and spell, as the development of both spoken and written language skills is closely linked. Conversely, children who have needs with speech and language development are at risk of having associated literacy needs.

Studies are now indicating the importance of visual verbal learning and the role of semantics in the development of mature reading skills. Poor reading comprehension is linked to limited listening span and a reduced ability to make semantic judgements. The morphological approach developed at Maple Hayes School in Lichfield is particularly successful in supporting pupils with this type of dyslexia (Peer & Reid, 2011).

Children with dyslexia often have impaired auditory processing skills and working memory deficits as a key feature of their dyslexia and tend to become more tired and frustrated than other children. Their attention must be maintained through interesting and varied instructional activities. Repetition of learning is also important and can be achieved by ongoing review.

In the literature, there is a broad range of opinion regarding what is involved in auditory processing. One auditory processing programme looks at the following six aspects of auditory processing:

- auditory discrimination;
- auditory memory;
- auditory perception;
- auditory association;
- auditory synthesis; and
- auditory comprehension.

Activities within the programme are arranged in order of progression, from the least difficult to the most difficult, so that each session builds on the previous one. The child is enabled to tackle gradually more difficult activities whilst still experiencing success at each level. However, because all children do not learn alike they cannot be taught alike, and therefore materials are selected based on the learning and instructional requirements of each individual. Each activity is presented in short, intensive periods of instruction. The activities are presented auditorily but worksheets are also included under each of these areas to take advantage of any strengths in visual processing that some children may have. The auditory/visual association provided by the worksheet activities is often essential for learning new concepts and language by children with limited auditory skills.

Fatima's story

Fatima was always a happy child but when she was about 2 years old I noticed that she wasn't putting words together as she should, and that I often couldn't understand her. She was referred to a speech and language therapist and received speech therapy on and off until she was 9 years old. She couldn't really talk in sentences and also found it hard to follow other people's conversation. Eventually, she was discharged from the speech and language therapy service, who more or less said that her very poor level of speech matched her 'cognitive abilities' – she was achieving all she was capable of.

She always struggled in school as she found it hard to follow the teacher, and when she was 5 years old I requested a statutory assessment. The local authority refused and I allowed myself to be reassured by the fact that she was still receiving speech therapy and hoped she would make progress. And she did, on and off; she worked so hard at school and at home where she tried to catch up with what she hadn't understood in class. She also found making friends very hard because she couldn't follow their conversations so became very isolated, and by the time she was 15 she came very close to a breakdown.

I had raised concerns with the school and the speech and language service on many occasions but had always been told 'she's just shy' or 'she's got learning difficulties' – finally, I had had enough and picked up the phone to a solicitor. I talked through the issues and sent some of the documents from Fatima's previous speech therapy and the solicitor advised me that we may have a chance of getting Fatima 'statemented'. We thought long and hard before employing the legal firm as it was very expensive, but because Fatima was already almost 16, we thought that we couldn't afford to make any mistakes as the process is pretty daunting. We raised the money (by remortgaging our house) and requested a statutory assessment. As part of that process, the solicitor recommended that we get professional reports carried out on Fatima, so we obtained reports from a speech and language therapist, an educational psychologist and a child psychiatrist. I still remember the emotion of finally having my worries confirmed and explained. Fatima was not just shy, she didn't have learning difficulties, she had severe speech and language needs and severe impairment of her auditory recall and speed of processing – no wonder she couldn't follow the teacher or keep up in class. Getting those reports was the best thing I ever did as it is so easy for a school to dismiss the worries of an 'anxious mum', but very hard for them to argue with an expert report.

The local authority refused to carry out a statutory assessment of Fatima but we appealed with the help of our solicitor and the LEA backed down at the last minute before the appeal. After the assessment they issued a Note-in-Lieu instead of a Statement – pretty worthless – so we had to appeal again, but this time the LEA didn't back down and we went to the tribunal. We were represented by a barrister, and our speech and language therapist and educational psychologist appeared as our witnesses. It was very daunting and stressful, but very reassuring to have a barrister and our experts there who knew our case inside out. The panel at the tribunal were fantastic, they were so clear on all the issues and so fair, that even if we had lost I could not have complained that we didn't get a fair hearing – but we won! The LEA was ordered to issue a Statement.

In the meantime, we had decided that there was no way Fatima could cope in a mainstream college or sixth form so took the decision to remortgage our house yet again and pay to send her privately to a specialist residential college. And when her GCSE results arrived she had obtained the magic '5 GCSEs at Grade C and above' despite all the odds – testament to her persistence and proof that she isn't hopeless academically, just severely disabled by her speech and language needs.

When the long-awaited Statement arrived from the LEA it didn't name the specialist college. It just said she could have speech therapy in a mainstream school with some one-to-one support from a learning support assistant. This would have been a disaster for Fatima – years of experience had taught us that she just can't cope with the type and speed of teaching in a mainstream school, and that she needs to be with pupils with similar issues so that she can finally fit in. We had to appeal yet again to try to get the LEA to fund Fatima at college for her final year – she is entitled to stay in school till the summer after her 19th birthday. Fatima had really settled in at the school and was much happier – just what you always dream of as a parent; although we missed her and were always worried about money, we knew that we had done the right thing.

Once again we had to produce more reports from our experts, with our third remortgage, this time to prove that the mainstream school 'named' in Part 4 of our Statement was unsuitable for Fatima, and that the specialist college was the right place for her. At this stage, the LEA still hadn't even got its own speech and language assessment done of Fatima – extraordinary when you consider that's her primary need! They seemed to be relying on the fact that the specialist college was 'too expensive' and that Fatima could manage in their mainstream school.

The LEA finally got a speech and language therapist to assess Fatima three weeks before the tribunal date! And on the last working day before the tribunal, at 5pm, after almost two years of fighting, our barrister contacted us to tell us the LEA had offered a 'part-funding deal' – basically they would pay for Fatima to remain at college until she is 19, if we pay a small part towards it. They had finally admitted that Fatima did need the education and integrated therapies only available at a specialist school!

We're so relieved it's over. The process is incredibly stressful and makes you very cynical – there is no incentive for the education authority to do the right thing by your child; by constantly refusing to assess, or to issue a Statement, or to name the school you know is the right one for your child, they shorten the time they may actually have to pay out to give the child a proper education, without fear of penalty. I'm told that the SEN system has been improved in recent years – well, I'd have hated to see it before. No one can quite believe how hard we've had to fight for what should be a basic right – an appropriate education for our child – and no one can quite believe that we won't get any of our legal costs back, or the fees we've already paid for a school the LEA now admits is the appropriate place for Fatima.

The advice I would give to any parent worried about their child is: trust your instincts, not the school's reassurances; get proper assessments done early, even if they seem expensive – they are money well spent; then be clear on what you're hoping to achieve. You've got to weigh up the very great costs of the legal process (each tribunal has cost us between £10,000 and £15,000 in legal and expert fees, though this would have been far less had we taken our own case without solicitors) against what your child is going to get out of it – how old is your child, how many years' education does (s)he have left? Does (s)he need a special school? Could your money be better sent buying in some therapies privately? Take early advice from a solicitor or one of the specialist charities. And don't give up – if you have a strong case and get the right help, the tribunal itself is very fair and you will be listened to.

Gabriel's story

Gabriel and his brother, Harvey, are both dyslexic. There is a strong family history of dyslexia on both sides of their family. Gabriel was born almost 10 weeks prematurely by Caesarean section as he was not growing in utero. At birth, he weighed 2lbs 1½ ozs and was on a ventilator and under a heat lamp for several weeks. At 1 week old, Gabriel had mucous in his throat and at 2–3 weeks he had septicaemia. Gabriel remained in hospital for 10 weeks and was discharged home when he reached 5lbs in weight. During the first 10 weeks of life he experienced three blood transfusions. Gabriel had many hospitalizations until the age of 5 with breathing difficulties. He is allergic to dairy products, citrus and egg. Even soya milk causes diarrhoea and he had to be fed using Aptomil and is now on a specialized diet. Gabriel likes to eat but is still very slow and messy. He has powdery enamel on his teeth. Gabriel was a late walker and did not crawl; he presents with a number of occupational therapy difficulties, all of which are combining to hinder his performance both at home and at school. Gabriel has made progress due to the occupational therapy intervention he has received, but he has remained behind the expected level for his peers, especially when time and pressure are applied to the situation. Sports coaching has also helped his coordination.

Concerns first arose at the beginning of Year 1 at school as Gabriel experienced many ear infections and at 5–6 years of age he needed grommets. When he was 8, Gabriel was diagnosed with Irlen Syndrome and was prescribed yellow lenses for a short period. Gabriel has difficulty in getting to sleep in the evening and is often not asleep until 10pm and then has to be woken in order to be ready for school at 7am.

Gabriel gets on well with adults. He enjoys cooking and is improving at it, he also likes playing on the computer and watching television especially 'Johnny English', 'Shrek', 'Harry Potter' and 'Star Wars'. When younger, Gabriel had problems with being still, hyperactivity, sleeping, concentrating, toilet training, eating and tantrums.

Gabriel was looked after by a childminder from 1 to 3 years of age. He then had two years of attending a nursery before attending school. Gabriel was diagnosed with dyslexia at the Dyslexia Institute when he was 7 years of age. At the end of Year 2, he was achieving at below average levels for reading, writing, spelling, comprehension and maths and his first Statement of Special Educational Needs was issued. Gabriel had special educational needs arising from his literacy and coordination needs plus short-term auditory and visual memory and fine motor skills.

Gabriel's difficulties can be ascribed to developmental dyspraxia with the coexistence of dyslexia, dyscalculia and dysgraphia. The Statement provided advice and support from an educational psychologist, and a cognition and learning specialist teacher. Gabriel also received 4–6 professional occupational therapy sessions per term to implement and monitor a programme set up by the school.

He transferred to a small independent school as a result of his emotional state and lack of progress at his previous school, even with five months' extra dyslexia tuition. Gabriel's reading had improved since he changed schools but he did not receive any occupational therapy there. Gabriel only had one friend at his previous school but had more friendly peers at his new school. The independent educational psychologist commissioned by his parents considered that Gabriel was not making adequate progress; he had severe dyslexia, dyspraxia and dyscalculia, poor phonological awareness and extremely poor rapid naming.

Gabriel had a growing awareness of the disparity between his high level thinking and his extremely low literacy skills. The EP recommended daily 1-hour sessions in literacy using a structured sequential multisensory programme delivered by a teacher who is dyslexia trained. In addition, she considered that Gabriel needed daily sessions of 45 minutes for specific numeracy tuition delivered in a small group, a learning skills programme and memory skills training, touch typing and all subject lessons to be taught by teachers who have received dyslexia training. In her view, Gabriel needed to attend a specialist dyslexia school in a class of no more than eight children.

Gabriel is motivated to want to read. Despite the effort involved he always tries his best and tackles new tasks with a positive attitude. Regarding speech and language development, Gabriel did not say his first words until he was 2 years of age, which was attributed to his history of ear infections. He had never been referred for speech and language therapy or an assessment. Following a successful SENDIST hearing, Gabriel was placed in a specialist residential school for pupils with severe dyslexia.

Harvey's story

Harvey is Gabriel's younger brother. He was born two weeks early by Caesarean section weighing 6.7 lbs, and there were no problems during the pregnancy. After Harvey was born, he had what was described as 'breast milk jaundice'. He was also very jumpy; lots of blood tests were done but these found nothing. Harvey is allergic to dairy and soya but he is mostly OK with them in small doses now. He walked independently at 11 months. Harvey is small in comparison to his peers, but has always been boisterous and plays roughly. He had strong left hand dominance from an early age. Harvey has had lots of ear infections; the hospital assessed him twice and told his that nature had sorted the problem out. Harvey is described by his parents as a reasonably good-natured child who has always been very loud. He enjoys fishing and is interested in all sports. He is beginning to enjoy his own company occasionally. Difficulties had been noted in relation to tantrums, concentration and discipline. Socially, Harvey was able to interact in a group but he did not seem to have strong relationships. He gets on well with his brother and adults and missed his brother when he went away to school. Harvey enjoys DIY, Cubs and judo.

Harvey was often frustrated and very angry; he had difficulty making choices and withdrew if he didn't understand something. He could not manage money. Harvey was reluctant to try new things; he lacked confidence and needed a lot of encouragement to attend things like judo which he does enjoy. Reasonable requests can lead to explosive outbursts.

Harvey attended his local school without a Statement, and his parents wanted him to attend the specialist dyslexia school with his brother as they could see the progress Gabriel was making, not only with his reading and writing but also in his self-esteem and condfidence. Harvey's parents considered he was really struggling at school, he could not read his own writing, his reading was behind his peers despite two years' specialized teaching, and phonics and spelling were a real problem. Harvey had issues with self image and, despite the effort he was putting in, he was not rewarded with results he could appreciate. Harvey's parents had been through the same issues with his brother who had become very distressed; they did not want this repeated with Harvey. Harvey completed a nightly 10-minute reading programme, *Toe by Toe*, which was suggested by the Dyslexia Research Institute. He attended a private dyslexia teaching session on Tuesday lunchtimes and received nightly homework from this. He had participated in a phonics programme initiated by his school. Harvey appeared to be able to retain more information when he wrote it down; however, he had difficulty with writing. The SENCO reported that Harvey was performing below average at reading, writing and spelling and was average at speaking and listening, maths, comprehension, science, history, geography and French.

Harvey was on School Action Plus. This stated his primary need was in literacy, reading and writing. Harvey received the following provision in his local mainstream school:

- 1:1 4 times weekly – building sight vocabulary; continue with remaining Year 2 and Year 3 words.
- 1:1 4 times weekly – daily reading to help build phonological awareness and increase reading for meaning.
- 1:1 4 times weekly – *Toe by Toe* – to be able to recall and use initial and final sounds in reading and writing.
- 1:20 4 times weekly – phonic development and spelling.
- 1:3 once a week – Teodorescu Programme – to be able to form letters correctly when writing.

The independent educational psychology assessment and report stated that Harvey was a very bright child who has moderate dyslexia and poor motor coordination, extremely poor working memory, poor phonological memory and poor rapid naming skills. His self-esteem was 'much lower than average', and his emotional response to failure was a concern. He was struggling in school – to the extent that he was being forced to attend by his parents – as he saw the gap widening between his functioning and that of his peers.

His brother was so distressed by similar difficulties that he carried out self harm of a serious nature. It was the view of his parents that Harvey's emotional state was similar to that of his brother; Harvey had already tried to self harm. The EP report also stated that Harvey's overall cognitive ability, as evaluated by the Wechsler Intelligence Scale for Children could not easily be summarized because his verbal reasoning abilities were much better developed than his non-verbal reasoning abilities. His reasoning abilities on verbal tasks were in the superior range; however, his non-verbal reasoning was significantly lower.

Harvey's abilities to sustain attention, concentrate and exert mental control were a weakness relative to his non-verbal and verbal reasoning abilities. Harvey's ability to process visual material quickly was also a weakness relative to his verbal and non-verbal reasoning ability. The EP recommended that Harvey see a child psychiatrist and be monitored closely. She also recommended he saw a speech and language therapist and an occupational therapist, and that he should receive more specialist dyslexia teaching in literacy and numeracy.

When Harvey was first learning to speak, he often missed the beginning of words, it was as if his ears were blocked intermittently and new words he encountered during this phase did not have beginnings. Harvey can now articulate, but using visual clues and an interactive style to communicate. He struggles to describe an activity he has done without any prompts. Harvey's parents were concerned about his inability to find the word he needs to say and his struggle to string words together when he is thinking. They were also concerned that Harvey has trouble with pronunciation despite having said the word correctly immediately before. Ironically, Harvey was put on the gifted and talented register for public speaking by his mainstream primary school just before the SENDIST hearing.

The tribunal hearing was attended by a speech and language therapist, EP, Harvey's parents and their representative (a specialist education law solicitor), the LEA and the LEA educational psychologist and the deputy head of the school Harvey attended. The LEA considered that Harvey was making progress but not as quickly as the parents would wish. Harvey's parents pointed out that all the educational psychologists who had assessed Harvey considered that he is a very able child with a low level of functioning. He is bright, but he is not going to reach his potential. The school and parents both put in extra provision but, despite this, his attainments remained low. There were specific needs which were not addressed at all. Under time pressure, his difficulties were worse. His self-esteem had been adversely affected. The tribunal panel agreed that Harvey needed a statutory assessment and a Statement of SEN.

Following the SENDIST order, a proposed Statement was issued. The Statement made provision for five hours teaching assistant support per week to support Harvey's self-esteem and confidence, a literacy programme and social skills/emotional literacy support. Harvey's parents appealed the contents of Parts 2, 3 and 4 of this Statement as although this was an improvement in provision they believed that he needed a specialist school placement and integrated SALT. Following a second SENDIST hearing, Harvey joined his brother, Gabriel, at the specialist residential school for pupils with dyslexia and is at last happy and making progress.

Dyscalculia

Many children have difficulty learning mathematics for a variety of reasons. Not all of these students have dyscalculia. However, there are some basic areas of mathematical activity in everyday life that may indicate a dyscalculic tendency if a person persistently finds it difficult and frustrating.

In very simple terms, analogous to dyslexia – which is dysfunction in the reception, comprehension, or production of linguistic information – dyscalculia can be defined as the dysfunction in the reception, comprehension, or production of quantitative and spatial information. Dyscalculia is a condition that affects the ability to acquire arithmetical skills. Dyscalculic learners may have difficulty understanding simple number concepts, lack an intuitive grasp of numbers, and have problems learning number facts and procedures. Even if they produce a correct answer or use a correct method, they may do so mechanically and without confidence.

Dyscalculia is a collection of symptoms of learning disability involving the most basic aspect of arithmetical skills. On the surface, these relate to basic concepts such as telling the time, calculating prices and handling change, and measuring and estimating things such as temperature and speed. Dyscalculia is an individual's difficulty in conceptualizing numbers, number relationships, outcomes of numerical operations and estimation – what to expect as an outcome of an operation. Dyscalculia manifests in a person as having difficulty:

- mastering arithmetic facts by the traditional methods of teaching, particularly the methods involving counting;
- dealing with exchange of money – handling a bank account, giving and receiving change;
- learning abstract concepts of time and direction/schedules, telling and keeping track of time, and the sequence of past and future events;
- acquiring spatial orientation/space organization/direction, easily disoriented (including left/right orientation), trouble reading maps, and grappling with mechanical processes;
- learning musical concepts, following directions in sports that demand sequencing or rules, and keeping track of scores and players during games such as cards and board games;
- following sequential directions – sequencing (including reading numbers out of sequence, substitutions, reversals, omissions and doing operations backwards), organizing detailed information, remembering specific facts and formulas for completing their mathematical calculations.

Dyscalculia can be quantitative, which is a difficulty in counting and calculating; or qualitative, which is a difficulty in the conceptualizing of mathematics processes and spatial sense; or mixed, which is the inability to integrate quantity and space.

Concluding remarks

Many schools are now dyslexia friendly and have teachers, advisory or on staff who have responsibility for organizing the support and additional teaching children with specific learning disabilities need. These interventions are effective and appropriate for the majority of children but they will not work for all children. Those with severe needs require a whole school multi-sensory approach.

7 Speech, language and communication needs: Hearing, understanding and talking

Introduction

This chapter features personal stories about Ida, Jensen, Keenan, Lennox and Milo. These children all have speech, language and communication needs (SLCN). Ida also has ASC. Jensen had complex communication needs which affected his behaviour as a young child. Keenan is severely dyspraxic. It had been assumed that he had general learning difficulties because he could not communicate properly or clearly and that his language was in line with his cognitive ability, and he was therefore not a high priority for speech and language therapy. Lennox and Milo both have SLCN as a result of their congenital deafness. Both have a cochlear implant; Lennox also has ADHD. It is also clear from these stories that, although SLCN are very commonly found in children, they are often misdiagnosed and children are placed in schools for children with moderate learning difficulties or autistic spectrum disorder on some occasions because that is where the SALT provision is rather than because that is the most appropriate placement for the child.

Speech, language and communication needs (SLCN)

Three children in every primary school classroom has SLCN (Law et al., 2000). SLCN is the most common type of special educational need (SEN) in children below 7 years of age and half of all children with SEN have SLCN (The Lamb Inquiry, 2009). The Bercow Report (2008) identified five key themes:

- Communication is crucial.
- Early identification and intervention are essential.
- A continuum of services designed around the family is needed.

- Joint working is critical.
- The current system is characterized by high variability and lack of equity.

Communication disabilities can leave children isolated, frustrated and excluded, and can also have a profound effect on their confidence and self-esteem. Speech and language needs present a huge problem. If children cannot develop language and communication, their chances of learning and achieving literacy or numeracy targets or developing life skills are negligible. This in turn can lead to disruption of their social and academic progress. They may have difficulty in understanding what is said to them (as well as what is said around them), in expressing needs, thoughts and feelings, in developing vocabulary and using well-formed sentences.

The learning context of the school is different from the learning context of the home. The two provide a contrasting set of opportunities in which the child can learn. Some of these contrasts are obvious: in school, children spend a lot of their time learning in groups. Adult:child interaction is perhaps less intimate than at home, with children making demands on peers more of the time and learning from each other. Therefore, a child with SLCN is likely to have less in-depth interaction with peers than that enjoyed by other children. Current thinking also highlights the importance of taking peer relationships into consideration when deciding on education placements for a child with SLCN.

Ida's story

Ida's story will be all too familiar to so many parents who will have gone through the same emotional stress of being forced to place their child in a wholly unsuitable school due to a flawed tribunal hearing. It took a long judicial review process, and an even longer compilation of evidence towards a second tribunal hearing to prove that her needs were not being met by the authority concerned, so that around three years of her education were lost.

Her needs centred around speech and language and ASC, whilst in general she demonstrated very good learning ability. The LEA, however, persuaded the tribunal that her needs could be met in a unit for children with autism in a school for children with moderate learning needs. All of our evidence that she needed intensive therapies was upheld by the initial tribunal, and was not challenged as such, but the major flaw was that the authority claimed that they could easily buy in the therapy, and the panel accepted this.

However, once she was placed into their school, they immediately declared that it would take many months to provide such specialist therapy, and were subsequently in breach of the law for the same number of months. Next, they managed to narrowly avert a judicial review hearing by providing some therapy, but worst of all was their decision at the next annual review to drop all of this provision, without giving any real evidence as to why. In this way, they demonstrated a complete and utter contempt for the tribunal's order.

Naturally, this action gave us grounds to open another long appeal process, but it is important not to underestimate the impact that all of this had on her and ourselves. Instead of receiving the vital support which her Statement defined, she was effectively languishing in the wrong environment, stuck in an ASC unit with non-verbal and unsuitable peers for almost two years. We were unable to work properly with the school staff, as we were effectively doing all we could to build up a case to remove her, whilst most of our free time was spent poring over documents, writing long reports, and logging every detail to create the evidence to prove what was at fault and turn things around. Our social life as a family was affected, since we were wholly preoccupied by the appeal, and everything else came second. Most importantly of all, her needs were being neglected much of the time still further, as we were putting so much time and energy into the appeal.

In the midst of this, it did become clear that we must focus more on her abilities and strengths, and it was at this point that she started to learn the piano. We had always been aware that she was musical, and fortunately she soon showed that, with much patience and hard work, she had a strong aptitude for it, and it has since changed her life dramatically. It has become the most important therapeutic activity in her life, and changed the way our whole family lives. By the time we had compiled a very long case statement towards our second hearing, she had been playing for one year, and had already achieved Distinction at Grade One. This became a highlight of our supporting evidence to finally disprove the authority's claim that she had MLD, and not long after this they were forced to put into writing that their school could not meet her needs. They eventually agreed to our choice of provision, but continued to delay things for a further few weeks, mainly by not being cooperative in writing our working document for as long as possible.

In the end, the only way we were able to prevent further procrastination was to threaten them that we would still go to the hearing.

Ida has now been at the preferred school for a little over two years. It is a small, specialist school for children with severe speech, language and communication needs, and she has done very well there. Whilst her difficulties remain severe, she is a model student who loves going to school, works hard, and enjoys all sorts of activities with her peers. Most importantly, she responds well to the therapy and is progressing, and we feel reassured that the long fight to obtain that all-important suitable provision for her was and has been fully vindicated.

It has been especially liberating to have been able to put away our bundles, and concentrate on parenting and on helping her, and developing a positive and close relationship with the school staff and other children and their families. Most encouraging of all is her continuing talent for and development of her music. In the same period of time, she has now passed Grades Two, Three, Four and Five, all with Distinction, and has had great success at many music festivals, as well as taking part in a master class and an orchestral workshop. She also studies ballet, and as a family we attend many music recitals and performances. Although she is still only 10 years old, we feel that all of this is very encouraging for her future prospects and her self awareness, especially when we think back to where we were before, and how so much time was lost.

Jensen's story

Jensen was a healthy baby who appeared to develop normally until he was 8 months old when he became ill with measles. Jensen had started to babble and was very vocal, but the single word stage just did not come, and as he was growing and meeting his milestones in every other way, we did not realize that there was a problem.

When Jensen was 1, we still could not recognize any intelligible words and became a little concerned as this was very different from our other child who had been articulate from a very young age.

By the age of 2, Jensen was doing most things that other 2-year-olds do except for language. He was very communicative, had reciprocal eye contact and would chatter away in his own little language which was expressive and tuneful. He appeared to have an understanding of what was going on around him and could follow simple instructions.

However, I was a little concerned. I felt that something wasn't quite right. My health visitor referred Jensen for a hearing test, just to rule out hearing problems as a result of the measles. He passed the test with flying colours and everybody continued to reassure me that everything was fine. I began to feel that I was being paranoid.

We began to notice a change in Jensen's behaviour. He became very frustrated and angry when he could not express himself and he had difficulty socializing with children his own age. He was not good at sharing and would lash out if another child attempted to take one of his toys. We started to see patterns of repetitive play. It was during this time that we really became concerned, especially as the health visitor referred him to speech and language therapy.

Initially we attended group sessions for the therapy, but Jensen found this difficult and would not cooperate so I was given instructions on activities to improve attention and listening and we had an individual session with the SALT every six weeks. Every day I would play with Jensen and try to engage him in activities to improve these skills. I tried to make it fun and engage his sister as well, but she quickly became bored.

We were introduced to the Early Years Advisory Teacher who arranged for Jensen to have 1:1 support at the local village playgroup. During this time, it became clear to us and to the professionals involved that Jensen did not have delayed language but a more complex communication disorder. The playgroup was linked to the local primary school, and as our daughter was already there I made enquiries about the support that might be available for Jensen. The head teacher told me that he would be better off in a specialist school. This was a devastating blow, as we had never envisaged that he would not be able to attend mainstream school. I was so alarmed by his head's response that I decided to look at other mainstream schools in the area, and we were very fortunate to find a head teacher who was very sympathetic and who offered Jensen a place in a mainstream nursery. He also encouraged us to get an assessment from the local authority.

We were successful in obtaining a Statement of Special Educational Needs for Jensen, which identified him as having difficulties with communication. This secured some 1:1 support and block sessions of speech and language therapy. However, time marched on and we agreed with the head teacher that Jensen would benefit from attending a school that had a speech and language unit. We made an application to the LEA but were refused a place on the grounds that Jensen's difficulties were too complex or could not be met in the language unit. We were now at a loss as to what to do.

Jensen was then 5 and had been assessed by four educational

psychologists, one community paediatrician and three different SALTs. As he was clearly having difficulty integrating, we were encouraged to consider a specialist autistic unit even though he did not have a diagnosis of autism! The LEA then suggested that an EBD unit could offer the support he needed but, having visited, we disagreed with their decision.

Jensen was now displaying some aggressive and disruptive behaviour which we believed was due to his frustration with not understanding or being able to express himself. We felt that the LEA was focusing on the behavioural aspects of his communication difficulties rather than the underlying problem and they would not acknowledge that they did not have appropriate resources to meet Jensen's specific needs.

It was at that point that I engaged the help of AFASIC (the Association For All Speech-Impaired Children) and started to investigate independent out-of-county provision. We felt very let down by the 'system', especially as this was around the time the government was implementing inclusive education. It was clear to us that the LEA could not provide a school that would accommodate Jensen's needs, but eventually the LEA offered him a place at a mainstream school on the other side of the county which had a newly-developed language base. We reluctantly accepted this offer as it was clear the LEA was not going to consider our suggestion of an independent placement. The school quickly recognized that this was not an appropriate placement for Jensen, and whilst they did their best to support him it clearly put a strain on their resources. Jensen spent a year there but he had little opportunity to integrate into the main school and spent most of his time on his own with the teacher or the language base.

After several independent assessments and paying for legal support we sought a judicial review on the grounds that the LEA had breached the code of conduct for SEN as they had failed to deliver appropriate support within the given timeframes. Jensen missed out a whole academic year before his situation was resolved. This caused him a lot of unnecessary distress, as he was socially isolated and did not have the opportunity to learn. It also caused a lot of stress to us as a family as we spent copious amounts of time fighting for Jensen's rights, which put us under huge emotional and financial pressure. Looking back, I feel saddened that we spent so much time agonizing and arguing over what was going on that we missed out on quality time with both of our children.

Nearly three years after starting the process, we finally secured Jensen a place, with LEA agreement, at an out-of-county specialist residential primary school for children with SLCN. We were delighted that we had succeeded in finding a school that matched our son's needs, but it was a traumatic time for us as we had not anticipated just how much we would miss him, and we certainly did not realize the impact that this would have on his sister. It was an incredibly difficult decision to send our small child to a boarding school at such a young age and one that I never thought that we would have to make. However, this school had a family support worker who was a tremendous emotional support to us and who helped us adapt to our new lifestyle.

On joining the school at almost 7, Jensen was described as 'a confused and angry little boy with low self esteem'. Within three months he had become a different child. He had settled well, he was joining in with his peers and he was beginning to trust the adults around him.

Jensen continued to make steady but slow progress throughout his five years at primary school, it having become clear that he had significant complex needs with both expressive and receptive language. It was at this point that we realized he would probably have to spend his entire education in specialist schooling.

When it came for time for Jensen to leave, we were worried that the LEA would see how much progress he had made and would want to provide support for him in mainstream. As it turned out, there was no question of him returning to mainstream and we were delighted when he was accepted by a specialist out-of-county residential secondary school for pupils with SLCN and the transition from primary to secondary went ahead without any problem.

Jensen spent five happy years there. He continued to make steady progress; he made friends and grew in confidence. He became interested in sports and represented the school at football, swimming and athletics. We were so proud when we attended the leaver's assembly and listened to him stand up in front of everyone and deliver a speech. He was full of confidence and had everyone laughing – a far cry from the little boy who would sit on the sidelines.

Jensen left secondary school a happy, confident teenager who loves being with his friends. He has a wicked sense of humour, is an enthusiastic sportsman and has 5 GCSEs. Initially, after the GCSEs the LEA wanted Jensen to go to a local mainstream college, and although this may be an option in the future we argued that he was not yet ready for mainstream. We felt strongly that Jensen needed time to mature and to continue to have intensive integrated support to help him consolidate what he had already learned. After much negotiation, and again having to seek legal support, we were successful in obtaining a place for him at a specialist residential out- of-county FE Centre for pupils with SLCN.

Jensen is happier than he has ever been. He has a peer group with whom he is very popular, he is travelling independently and takes part in football training with one of the local teams. He socializes in the local community and is a regular at the British Legion where he plays pool and watches football. He has joined a local athletics club and has represented his school in athletics championships. He is also learning to drive.

Most young people reach the age of 18 and decide they want to leave home. For Jensen, it is the opposite. Having spent all of his school life in residential settings Jensen is happy to come home. It feels right that he should be doing this as he has missed out on normal family life and needs to be part of it again. No doubt we will have a few ups and downs but I am sure that we will learn to adjust and adapt.

We are now exploring the possibilities of a local college placement. Jensen has seen some courses in construction and he is also going to look for part-time work. He also hopes to join a local football club and fulfil his dream of playing in a competitive league.

We now understand the extent of Jensen's communication problems and can see that he will have these needs for the rest of his life. Looking back at the choices we made and the problems we had, I am convinced that we did the right thing. Would we have done things differently had there been appropriate local provision? Probably not. Now that we are coming to the end of Jensen's school years I cannot see that things have changed much. There may be more schools in some areas with specialist units and more children may be getting some help, but I still think that children like Jensen need specialist support that is just not available in mainstream school.

Our son has grown into a kind, caring and charming young man and we are extremely proud of his achievements, all of which would not have been possible without the support of the dedicated staff at the specialist schools and FE centre and the support of AFASIC.

Dyspraxia

Dyspraxia is a specific learning difficulty (SpLD) so it does not affect overall intelligence or ability but just particular aspects of development. The Dyspraxia Foundation defines developmental dyspraxia as 'an impairment or immaturity of the organization of movement. It is an immaturity in the way that the brain processes information, which results in messages not being properly or fully transmitted. The term 'dyspraxia' comes from the word 'praxis', which means 'doing, acting'. Dyspraxia affects the planning of what to do and how to do it. It is associated with problems of perception, language and thought'.

Keenan's story

When we came in for Keenan's independent speech and language therapy assessment, on the advice of a specialist education law solicitor, we were facing huge problems. It had never been explained to us or Keenan exactly what his difficulties and needs were, the LEA could not or would not see a way forward for Keenan, and would not provide any extra SALT or OT provision for him. It was like we were banging our heads against a brick wall. We knew that our 9-year-old son was in desperate need of help but we didn't know what to do for him or how to help him.

The independent SALT's detailed, professional, clear assessment of Keenan changed everything. It was like a beacon of light giving us clear, unbiased answers to all of our questions and giving Keenan so much more – the possibility of a secure and independent future. For the first time, we understood clearly what Keenan's needs were and that he was of average ability. If Keenan was placed in the right specialist setting, and provided with daily support and provision, he could make progress.

The SALT was also able to provide Keenan with vital weekly SALT sessions, as by this stage all NHS SALT had been withdrawn from Keenan within his mainstream setting because we had appealed to SENDIST. Indeed, the assessment was so clear and well presented that, upon its disclosure, together with the EP and OT assessments we had also obtained, the LEA, who had been previously vigorously defending our appeal, decided not to contest it. Keenan was awarded the protection of an amended Statement providing him with all of the support and provision we were requesting, and a placement at one of the country's leading specialist schools for children with speech, language and communication needs for one year, and what a difference a year can make.

Keenan is now a happy and confident child, who is starting to talk clearly and achieve the potential that he clearly has. At the end of Year 6, Keenan achieved Level 4 in his Science SAT, not bad for a child who was being graded on P scales in his local mainstream primary. Keenan still has a long way to travel but he now has the full support he needs to achieve his true potential.

Deafness

About 3 in every 1000 children are born deaf and 1 in 1000 of these is born with a severe or profound deafness. There are about 23,000 deaf children in the UK. Ninety percent (9 out of 10) of deaf children are born to hearing parents. People who suffer from profound hearing loss are very hard of hearing and rely mostly on lip-reading and/or sign language.

Deafness and speech development

The presence of deafness does not have a simple or well-defined influence on the speech of children. Its effects are extremely varied and are complicated by the results of widely differing approaches to intervention. Phonology cannot be isolated from the other sub-systems of language and, where intervention is considered, all language levels and their influence on one another must be taken into account. The early and consistent use of high quality amplification and auditory training or auditory-verbal training in order to make maximum use of residual hearing is vital. The extent of the effect of hearing loss on speech development is extremely varied, involving the difference of linguistic input, as well as the hearing loss itself. For many deaf speakers' reduction in auditory acuity is accompanied by an increased reliance on visual cues and lip-reading/speech-reading.

Signing

Whatever views are held on the merits and difficulties of using sign with deaf children, the fact remains that the highly variable linguistic experience that each approach makes available to deaf children is bound to have an important influence on their acquisition of speech and language.

Cochlear implants

A cochlear implant is a medical device that helps a person with severe to profound hearing loss to experience 'hearing'. It's designed to mirror the intricacies of natural hearing. In contrast to a hearing aid, which simply makes sounds louder, a cochlear implant takes the place of parts in the inner ear that are not working properly.

The cochlear implant has two basic pieces:

- The **processor** is the piece outside the body. It picks up sounds, processes them, and sends signals to the cochlear implant.
- The **implant** is inside the body. It is placed behind the ear during surgery. It receives signals and sends them to the hearing nerves, skipping over any non-working parts in the middle and inner ear.

Lennox's story

Lennox is profoundly deaf and has a cochlear implant. My overall impression of Lennox's speech is that he is currently largely unintelligible. An experienced listener could follow a known text with lip reading but not from an audio tape. Use of signed support speech does help Lennox's intelligibility currently in face-to-face communication. However, his speech intelligibility is already showing some signs of improvement, particularly for consonant sounds produced in the middle of words. In my opinion, because of Lennox's degree of hearing loss, he needs to be taught by qualified teachers of the deaf in all subject areas with whom tutorials should also be available. Lennox needs to be encouraged to develop his speaking and listening skills to the full to achieve his potential and take his place in society. Lennox needs to be taught in acoustically treated classrooms with networked computers (with hearing aid adaptors), teletext facilities and access to the internet. Teletext TV with radio aid links and whisper-quiet overhead projectors need to be used to promote effective listening skills and enable Lennox to interpret spoken language effectively. All these provisions need to be in addition to specialist speech and language therapy for Lennox to achieve maximum progress.

Lennox is an only child and his parents are divorced. He was born two weeks late by emergency Caesarean section, weighing 9lbs 12ozs. Lennox's vision is reported to be brilliant and his motor milestones were normal. He was referred for a hearing test, aged 3 months and diagnosed at 8–9 months with profound bilateral sensori-neural deafness. Lennox initially wore post-aural hearing aids for 18 months and then body-worn aids for 18 months. A cochlear implant was implanted into his left ear when he was 4½ years of age and he was seen fortnightly by the cochlear implant team for nine years post implant.

Lennox's general health is good. By 8 years of age, his behaviour had not improved and his parents were advised to see a geneticist. Lennox was assessed for Oppositional Defiance Disorder and ADHD. Methylphenidate had an immediate effect. Lennox is monitored for his severe ADHD.

Lennox went to nursery at 3 years of age with a full time 1:1 teaching assistant and a teacher of the deaf visiting daily. On school entry, he attended a mainstream school with special provision for hearing impaired children. Lennox had additional teaching from a teacher of the deaf for one hour per day from reception to Year 3. Lennox then went to his local village school for Years 4–6, with a teacher of the deaf visiting for one hour per day to work on maths, science and English but he was was disapplied from SATS.

Lennox is now at secondary school and is very popular and outgoing. He has a full-time teaching assistant and spends six hours per week with a teacher of the deaf. Lennox is good at maths, design technology, ICT and sport and has a passion for cars. He is receiving additional teacher of the deaf tuition at home on Saturdays for reading, using Rebus symbols and Widgit software. Lennox has weekly speech and language therapy on his Statement. He receives fortnightly therapy from the NHS speech and language therapist, and did have fortnightly therapy from a specialist speech and language therapist from the cochlear implant team. The LEA then funded fortnightly independent speech and language therapy. Lennox is fortunate that weekly SALT has continued throughout his secondary years to age 19 and he has been supported by a hearing impaired unit and TAs who go with him into mainstream lessons, but his progress remains slow.

Lennox is now a young adult of 19 years but he is still functioning linguistically at approximately age 6–7 level. Compared to other young people of the same age, his communication remains very poor in both spoken and written forms due to his ADHD, ODD, profound deafness and language needs. He has successfully integrated into his year group. He has taken on key roles in both the Physical Education and Design and Technology departments during his time in 6th form and is part of the after-school cleaning team. Lennox has achieved a place at college to study furniture making and installation. We are all very proud of him.

Milo's story

Our second child, Milo, was born a beautiful, contented baby and a welcome addition to our family. As the months rolled by, we became unsure that he was able to hear properly, but felt reassured that he passed both his 8-

and 15-month hearing tests. I recall the health visitor saying that she was certain that Milo could hear but that he wouldn't play the 'listening game'. Either way, she felt sure that any hearing problem he may have would not affect his speech. How shocked we were to find out that he is profoundly deaf. After the shock came the sense of grief as we wondered what would become of him. Shortly after, I enrolled on a British Sign Language course and BSL became Milo's only method of communication until he was 4½ years old. We decided that Milo should have a cochlear implant and he was implanted. He also received follow-up care and speech and language therapy from the implant centre. This rehabilitation period only lasted just over a year and we were then left with a fight to get speech and language therapy for Milo.

The Advisory Teacher of the Deaf told us that deaf children were unable to receive this therapy as there was no-one trained to work with deaf children. Whilst trying to get help from the local authority, we decided that we needed to find a speech and language therapist immediately. We took Milo to a speech and language therapist for assessment and started paying for private therapy. Not only did Milo receive the help he desperately needed, but I became more knowledgeable and confident to take on the LEA to challenge the wording of the Statement. We prepared a watertight case, our SLT wrote a comprehensive report and this was accompanied by reports by the implant team and another speech and language therapist. We got to four days before the SEN tribunal and the LEA gave in. They agreed to fully fund Milo's therapy to be delivered by the independent SLT.

The SLT had given us facts, figures and warned us of the loopholes; the knowledge she armed us with was definitely a vital key to our success. To date, Milo still receives SLT and next year's Statement has been approved without change to the provision. Milo's speech is now intelligible and he has gained confidence to use his voice even with strangers. His chosen method of communication is now oral; however, he does still rely on sign language for receptive clarification.

Milo is a sporty young man; he loves to play football and he swims for the District Swimming Club and also competes with the British Deaf Swimming Squad. He is the holder of the British Deaf Swimming Record in all four strokes at 50 metres. He also loves cycling and often cycles about 20 miles on a Sunday morning with his dad. He hopes to complete his first triathlon very soon.

Concluding remarks

Many of these individuals have needs that persist well into adolescence and adulthood. Current thinking, however, indicates that associated psychiatric conditions are not caused by having SLCN but what happens to a child at school, what support they get and their rate of progress. There is a strong need for increased support for these young people and their families into adulthood, and specific education and speech and language therapy support being available at both primary and secondary levels.

8 Learning disability: Mild, moderate, severe or complex

Introduction

This chapter contains the personal stories of Nancy and Orlando. Their stories could have fitted into other chapters equally well, but they are here because they both have some degree of general cognitive learning disability in addition to their other diagnoses. Nancy is a child with selective mutism. Orlando has severe learning needs, ASC and challenging behaviour.

Selective mutism

Selective mutism is diagnosed when a child will speak to only a small number of people, in a particular environment or under a particular circumstance. A child who is selectively mute will usually speak to their immediate family members, in their home, when no-one else is present. The children usually struggle the most at school but these patterns vary on every selectively mute child. Selective mutism is a rare disorder which affects 2 to 18 children per 10,000. A diagnosis of selective mutism can vary depending on the source. Some researchers feel that after one month of mutism a diagnosis can be made, others feel six months is more appropriate to eliminate shyness or reluctance to talk. The symptoms are described as:

- consistent inability to speak in social situations despite speaking in other situations;
- unable to speak, causing interference with educational or occupational achievement or social communication;
- duration of mutism is at least one month;
- the mutism is not due to lack of knowledge of the language or social situation;
- there is not a more dominant communication or psychotic disorder.

Studies show that selective mutism is more common in girls than boys. Age of onset is thought to be from 3 to 5 years old. Selective mutism can be associated with other conditions such as anxiety, depression, enuresis, hyperactivity, encopresis (soiling), tics, obsessive-compulsive features, speech and/or language impairment, hypersensitivity and perfectionism.

A multi-modal approach to therapy for a child with selective mutism has been found the most successful. Behavioural methods are the most popular, working with a punishment and reward system, e.g. positive reinforcement for speaking and withholding reinforcement for mutism. A structured programme, Breaking down the Barriers, is based on behavioural therapy. A medicated drug that is popular in the USA, called selective serotonin reuptake inhibitors (SSRIs), is used for intervention with children who are diagnosed with selective mutism. Using a drug intervention has been most successful in children who have a multi-modal approach where sole approaches haven't succeeded.

Speech and language therapy needs to be individualized and child-centred and is most successful in children who have anxiety over their speech sounds. Self-modelling, where video tapes are altered to show the child speaking in an environment where they are usually mute, have been found successful. Involving the family with the child's therapy is essential when combined with the other methods.

Nancy's story

Nancy has one sister. There is no family history of any speech, language, communication, reading or writing difficulties. Scans during pregnancy showed a possible heart abnormality, but at birth Nancy had only a couple of small holes which closed without surgery. She was born one week overdue by emergency Caesarean section for foetal distress and weighed 2.57 kilograms (5lb 10.5oz). Nancy was in the special care baby unit and then transferred to Great Ormond Street Hospital after three days as she had dysmorphic features, poor feeding, dilated right heart chambers, dilated stomach and stenosis. Nancy suffers from hayfever but allergy tests have not shown what causes it. As a small baby, Nancy was admitted to hospital several times with chest infections.

Nancy hasn't really had any problems sucking, chewing or swallowing, but she doesn't eat anything that needs a lot of chewing and still occasionally chokes on foods. She made the transition to solids following extremely poor feeding with milk. A dietician saw Nancy as a baby and she now has a good and varied diet, although nothing chewy. Nancy has moderately severe developmental delay. During school term time, she suffers from constipation and is wet two or three times a day. She also stops talking. Nancy did not crawl, she bottom shuffled at about 2 years of age. She sat independently at about 1 year and walked independently at about 3 years of age. She had a rolator from about 2 years old and, prior to walking independently, would walk with minimal support, more for confidence than balance. She is still a bit unsteady on her feet and her fine motor skills are not great, either.

Nancy has 6-monthly appointments for glue ear. She has had glue ear and suffered from ear infections from birth to about age 5. Her hearing levels have varied but are apparently adequate to develop normal speech. She has had three sets of grommets between the ages of 13 months to 5 but these are now out. Nancy is long sighted and wears glasses. Nancy will talk to anyone and has no idea of stranger danger. At the moment, she wants to join in with other children's games but doesn't always understand how it works. If she is hurt by accident, she thinks it is deliberate and expects adult intervention to sort it out.

Nancy received speech and language therapy from about the age of 2. It seemed mostly to entail meetings with her father in which he was told that parents should talk to Nancy and make noises at her, which they knew and were doing anyway. Their other daughter was speaking reasonably clearly by 12 months, as a second child following one with special educational needs probably receives less attention. Nancy then went to a special school for children with severe and complex learning disabilities with a Statement of Special Educational Needs. Nancy's parents wanted to move her to a school for children with moderate learning disabilities, rather than the one for severe disabilities which was proposed by the LEA.

Nancy's parents appealed against Parts 2, 3 and 4 of the Statement with the help of IPSEA. The appeal in respects of Parts 2 and 3 were struck out. Regarding Part 4, Nancy's Statement specified the type of school, a special school catering for pupils with severe and complex learning difficulties, and the local authority's view was that a school of this type was appropriate for her. The authority opposed the naming of a moderate learning disability school on the grounds that Nancy's admission would be prejudicial to the efficient education of other pupils. The local authority considered that Nancy did not meet the admission criteria for a moderate learning disability school as she was banded as severe. Nancy's parents asked an independent speech and language therapist to assess their daughter. Nancy was cooperative and sociable throughout the session, even when she was really challenged by the tasks and reverted to whispering or sign. She could be coaxed to expand and extend her expression. Her play showed some well developed skills emerging and she demonstrated awareness and used social rules and skills. She had delayed development of understanding spoken language and of expression which was to be expected considering her medical diagnosis of global developmental delay. Despite this, Nancy was a successful communicator within environments where she felt comfortable and secure.

During the next academic year, her parents reported no dialogue with the LA. Nancy was going backwards at school and they decided to home educate her. Nancy learned to use the computer and could recognize 45 words. She was working on numbers to 30. She could order consistently to 13. However, Nancy's attainment depended on her concentration. She was still selectively mute and would not respond even to parents when under pressure of direct questioning. She attended an after-school club to integrate with her mainstream peers, and received therapy from an independent speech and language therapist for her selective mutism. A programme was being followed with a TA but this person left suddenly so the programme stopped.

Nancy was now dry at night as well as the day most of the time. Her constipation was much improved and she had been discharged by the paediatrician. An independent OT considered that it was evident that the level of therapeutic input to Nancy's education programme over the years had been inadequate and that she needed direct and indirect occupational and speech and language therapy. Nancy's selective mutism and related language/communication needs represented significant challenges to teaching and created the greatest barrier to learning.

Nancy needed to be able to communicate and socialize with people outside of her family and to function in environments outside of her home. The OT stated that consistency and continuity across school and care environments have very high importance in order to develop Nancy's potential, independence and daily living skills and function in a community. Nancy needs to develop communication skills so that she can communicate confidently across a range of social situations and contexts. Academically, her needs would be better met in a school for children with moderate learning needs and speech, language and communication needs.

As a result, Nancy's parents appealed the contents of her Statement of SEN. As the LEA would not contemplate the local school for pupils with moderate learning needs, Nancy's parents had her assessed at an out-of-county school which would mean that she would have to board. She was assessed in both one-to-one situations with specialist staff and in group situations with other pupils. The out-of-county residential specialist School for children with moderate learning needs combined with SLCN concluded that Nancy was very suitable for a place where they would be able to meet her functional, social and academic needs. It was in their view important that Nancy had the opportunity to transfer and generalize her learning by a general, holistic waking-day curriculum in a residential setting where she could be taught individually and in small groups. They offered her a boarding placement.

Unfortunately, the tribunal hearing did not go well. The combination of judge and LEA barrister was not a good one and the discussion of evidence went round and round in circles and took three days over several months to complete. The written decision did not agree with the parental team that Nancy needed to be placed in a school for children with moderate disabilities and communication needs, and agreed with the LEA's placement of Nancy in a school for children with severe and complex learning disabilities. The parents are now faced with an impossible dilemma. Do they:

- send Nancy to a school that they are not happy with and know will not be able to meet her needs and wait for her to fail again;
- face prosecution if they continue to home school her against the tribunal order;
- move house to see if they can find a more reasonable LEA with all the disruption that will have on the whole family, employment and their other child's schooling; or
- try to find alternative funding so that their daughter can go to the only school they have found that they truly believe can meet her needs and give her a chance of progress to reach her potential, whatever that is.

Orlando's story

Orlando was born by Caesarian section at 40 weeks gestation due to breech presentation. His birthweight was 8lbs. Orlando was a hungry baby but was often sick. Orlando has autism, severe learning difficulties, ADHD and challenging behaviour. He has two normally developing brothers. There is no known family history of speech, language, reading, writing, social skills or learning difficulties.

After his younger brother was born, when Orlando was 15 months, his behaviour became more noticeably different from other children of his age. He was assessed at a Child Development Centre (CDC), which recommended that their nursery nurse work with him at home in addition to the speech and language therapist seeing him at the CDC.

Orlando would only eat cheese and onion Pringles crisps (if unbroken), pot noodle, pasta, chips and, occasionally, sweetcorn. He did not eat any meat or fish, milk, fruit or other vegetables. He had a vitamin supplement daily and drank blackcurrant. Orlando was very overweight as a result (99.6th centile). He was always asking for food and always seemed to be hungry. He also suffered from constant diarrhoea and took medication for this regularly. Orlando has never slept well. He took Risperidone twice a day to calm his restlessness and Melatonin to help him sleep at night. Orlando was very noise sensitive and had sensory disintegration.

Orlando liked to be outside on long walks in the wood, otherwise he preferred to watch DVDs such as 'Cinderella'. He had a fascination with birds and feathers. Orlando could be loving and happy when he got his own way, but could also be aggressive and obstinate. Respite was increased to help his family cope with this increase in challenging behaviour.

Orlando attended a nursery for children with autism from the age of 3, and continued to have weekly music therapy.

At the age of 9, Orlando was still in nappies. He received a Statement of Special Educational Needs and continued to attend the ASC special school. He was there for several years but it was due to close and so Orlando had to move. He was in a class of three children and therefore he received 1:1 support all of the time. Most of the other pupils were going to a new special unit attached to a mainstream school but this was not appropriate for Orlando. His parents considered that the LEA would name a local SLD school for Orlando's future placement as it had a care home next door. Orlando was working at P3 for most subjects. The speech and language therapy service didn't work with children at Orlando's school, only with the staff. The school were working on PECS in a limited way at snack time. Orlando's NHS therapist considered that Orlando's needs could be met in the classroom by education staff working collaboratively on joint targets devised with a speech and language therapist, with the targets reviewed annually. She did not recommend any direct speech and language therapy. Orlando used *The Listening Programme* at school and was involved in sensory circuits. From reports, Orlando had made no progress in his communication skills over the previous year and his parents stated that this had been the case for 3–4 years.

Orlando's parents considered that for Orlando to make progress he needed to attend a specialist residential school, able to provide structured teaching on a waking day 52-week curriculum with opportunities for close supervision and leisure activities to enhance his development and chances of future independence. Orlando needed access to specialist support for complex needs, extended beyond the school day. They identified a school in the next county as the most suitable future educational placement for Orlando.

Orlando's parents were successful in their SENDIST appeal and Orlando attended a residential autism specific school for six months. This school provides specialist residential care and education for nine young people aged 11 to 19 who have autism and severe learning disabilities. Education and welfare provision is fully integrated and seamless, which means that from the time students wake up until the time they go to sleep in the evening they are engaged in productive activities that move their learning forward. After school, students have a wide choice of creative, leisure and home management activities, all of which complement and extend their learning in school. There is a strong emphasis on physical activity during the weekends and evenings. For the students, there are significant advantages to living and going to school in one location. The effectiveness of having the same management and staff teams bringing their skills together to support students throughout their waking day is the key to the students making progress. Care staff and teaching staff work together all the time and share staff training. Staff employ the same, consistent approach when implementing new learning and development in personal skills which spans both settings. The consultant therapists and psychologist work in the home setting as well as in school, enabling them to have a first-hand view of the students' needs throughout the waking day. Communication between the home and school is seamless. Staff at all levels meet on a daily basis to talk about the students and jointly work on care plans and education plans to ensure consistency. During his attendance at the school Orlando was toilet trained, he began communicating via a communication aid and PECS and he lost weight.

However, the LA successfully appealed the decision of the SENDIST panel in the High Court citing unreasonable use of public resources. The LA claimed that Orlando did not have an educational need for a residential placement, and if he did, he could be accommodated within county in order to give the family appropriate respite. Orlando had to leave his new school and become a Looked After Child in the care of the council even though there had never been a child protection issue raised and no concerns about his parents' love and care for him. He had a placement at a children's home with five young people in shared care. Orlando stayed at the children's home during the week and returned home for home visits every other weekend and during the school holidays.

During the day in term time, Orlando was educated in a new coeducational special school. The school catered for pupils between the ages of 3 and 19 years of age with severe or moderate learning difficulties. Some pupils had additional medical, physical or sensory impairments or emotional and behavioural difficulties.

Following his 14+ transition review, Orlando's Statement of Special Educational Needs was reissued. This allowed his parents the right of appeal to SENDIST, as they still considered that he needed a 52-week educational placement with a waking day curriculum. They wanted Orlando to return to the out-of-county specialist school as the residential placement is, in their view, an educational need.

I am delighted to say that when the LA costed Orlando's local provision of attendance at a special day school combined with shared care in a residential children's home, it was found to be more expensive than returning him. Therefore, the costing that they put to the High Court in order to win their appeal had been wrong and misleading. It cost Orlando's parents considerable financial and emotional hardship and stress and Orlando lost two full academic years. However, he has now settled back into the school where he wants to be and we wish him well for his future.

Concluding remarks

It is hard enough for any family to live and nurture a child with a complex mixture of learning needs. It is very expensive for a local education authority to educate these children. These two stories illustrate the importance of all statutory services communicating and working together with the families and joint funding placements that can meet all the needs of the child – health, education and social care. It would seem that sometimes LEAs make life harder for these families due to the constraints placed upon them and need to recognize the emotional and financial stress that their decisions have on the child and family forever.

Part III
The Future

9 The long view: Disabled children become adults

Introduction

Disabled children grow into adults and it is difficult for parents to imagine their young son or daughter at a different stage in life. The disabled child is often assigned a very specific role within the family and may therefore encounter additional obstacles on the road to adulthood. Parents are not necessarily helped with these transitions and, while being totally committed to helping their son or daughter to maximize their potential, find that there is no road map available for the journey.

Language and disability theory

The Medical Model of Disability views disability as synonymous with problem. Disabled people and the parents of disabled children are increasingly unhappy with this ideology which promotes the idea that impairment equates to deficit. In contrast, the Social Model of Disability views challenges experienced by people with impairments within their social context and poses the view that difficulties often arise by the way society functions (as a creation of non-disabled people). The Affirmative Model of Disability reminds us that disability is ordinary and impairment is not automatically undesirable – it is just a fact of life. We will all become disabled if we live long enough. The 'them and us' line, if it exists at all, has blurred and moveable edges.

Positioning disabled children as the negative other is something which may have life-long consequences in relation to the formation of healthy self-esteem. Parents who have contributed to this book are particularly concerned with not spoiling identity and with raising positive children. This chapter introduces ideas which will assist those stuck in the moment to take the longer view.

When a Russell Group university student was asked, 'How would you describe yourself?' and answered by saying 'I was a Special Needs Child', the double edged sword of disabled naming comes into sharp focus. Not all disabled people actively think about disability politics, of course, and therefore see language as a site of struggle.

Proponents of The Medical Model of Disability (regardless of whether they know the term) unselfconsciously use phrases like 'people with disabilities' or 'SEN children'. Charity, religious and tragedy models of disability are characterized by negative language antithetic to the notion of positive identity. A rejection of charity model thinking is illustrated by one mother's reaction to unwanted sympathy about her child's impairment, 'How dare you view my greatest achievement as a tragic event'. Parents of disabled children illustrated in previous chapters have multiple experiences of insensitive assumptions.

Viewing disability as a deficit within a person which needs fixing immediately positions the individual as 'other' in the sense of 'wrong' compared with the majority. Disability and impairment are not automatic bedfellows or interchangeable terms. The word 'impairment' refers to in-person characteristics such as having cerebral palsy. Consciously using the term 'disabled person' implies an understanding that external, not in-person, factors create disability. Impairment (for example, cerebral palsy) is a given, but disability occurs as a result of disabling environments.

Impairment does not have to be synonymous with disability but attitudinal and structural barriers will disable by limiting opportunity. Enormous barriers are currently being erected as a result of the current climate of spending cuts and reduction in services necessary to enable independent living. This fact is a huge threat to social justice and social inclusion of disabled people.

While structural barriers, such as stairs, are obvious, attitudinal barriers can limit life chances in ways which are not so easily visible. Teachers, parents, careers advisors and others can close the door to post-school education or employment unintentionally by making assumptions that the disabled person in transition will not be able to cope. Politicians can slash access to benefits, accessible transport, Access to Work funding and so on and, in so doing, catastrophically limit opportunities. It is easy to be bogged down with the here and now as a parent, and professionals may be used to working with children in a particular age range. However, disabled children do grow into adults and it is not possible to know what the aspirations of an 8-year-old will be when they are 21, whether they will grow up to be gay, how many children they might have, whether services they need will still exist, and so on.

We need to remain optimistic about these children as parental expectations may be massively exceeded. Parents may well have worked hard to limit their aspirations when their child received their diagnosis, only to then have to think again when the child learned to read, and again when the A level results came out, and so on and so on. While the point is made in preceding chapters that it is important to be realistic, realistically, when a child receives a diagnostic label we don't really know what this means.

Them and us

Disability terminology has the power to create a 'them and us' binary. The binary is central to notion of 'othering' in which 'the impaired' (them) are contrasted negatively with 'the dominant non impaired majority' (us). Disabled people, and parents of disabled children, increasingly reject the position of negative other. The following is a quote from a young adult which is reproduced anonymously with his permission:

'Having a diagnosis of Asperger syndrome as a child means that, as an adult, you can never interact normally with anyone ever again. It's because you know that, if they know, they will view everything you do through their knowledge that you have a diagnosis of AS. If they don't know, you worry that they will find out and react differently towards you'.

This highlights the feelings of alienation which a person can experience and which we all need to be aware of as our children develop into adults. The emerging political climate which portrays a negatively constructed other in the form of a disabled person who may not have equal access to a socially just infrastructure which will facilitate participation and inclusion is also concerning.

Legislation and inclusion

Disability is one of a range of protected characteristics covered within the Equality Act (2010) which also recognizes that people have multiple identities. Preceding equalities legislation described a positive duty to build good relationships between men and women, disabled and non-disabled people and ethnic groups. Despite the Equality Act, disablism is evident in language, culture and media. The Equality Act may be called upon to address concerns about limiting the opportunities of disabled people by reducing access to services necessary for social participation. The Equality Act requires leaders, governors and staff in post-school education to challenge oppression of marginalized groups, including disabled people. Widening Participation practitioners have a role to play.

The Equality Act aims to promote social inclusion. Inclusion equals belonging, the antithesis of 'othering'. Disabled students in post-school education have often reinvented themselves and experience a sense of reluctance about going near services that they associate with the negative SEN tag. Therefore, inclusive services, which diminish the requirement for a label may well be the way forward. Fear of discrimination is a reality for disabled college and university staff as well as students. Some with neurodiverse learning styles such as dyslexia or Asperger syndrome prefer to think in terms of neurological difference and reject the notion of disability. It is important to be sensitive to differences between and within individuals. Over time people change: change their minds, change direction and develop. Thinking in terms of the particular age group with whom one is professionally engaged, or one's child where they are now, is potentially limiting. Life is an exciting journey.

Concluding remarks

Disability is complex and socially constructed. Impairment does not necessarily equate to disability. If you are not a disabled person today it does not mean that you will not be a disabled person tomorrow. Identity is complicated and fluid. Impairment is only part of someone's identity. The Affirmative Model of disability reflects ordinariness of impairment. The Equality Act emphasizes inclusion, celebration of diversity and irradiation of barriers. Government spending cuts directly threaten the societal participation of disabled people and this is a very real concern. Parents of disabled children are operating in a complex and changing landscape. Professionals work with disabled people often within a narrow age band. Growth and development over time means that the life course of a disabled child is unpredictable. Parents are a constant. Professionals come and go. It is necessary to work together optimistically with the disabled person at the heart of the process. It is always essential to listen to that person and not to make any assumptions based on what you think they ought to do.

10
Celebration of strengths and ordinariness of impairment

Introduction

The fifteen personal stories in this book illustrate that many children with special educational needs have health and social care needs in addition to their educational needs. The common themes in the stories are that the children present with many different behavioural needs which often manifest in inflexibility, hyperactivity, defiance, disruptiveness, disobedience and rigidity. Parents find the hardest things to deal with are lack of communication and lack of sleep. Parents are therefore stressed and worried and exhausted but tell us there is no consistent respite. There may be financial worries, especially if the family has undertaken to instruct representatives, and especially if several SENDIST or court hearings occur. These families have lots of appointments, with lots of different professionals who change frequently and do not always communicate or work well together so that parents' concerns are dismissed as them being anxious. Local authorities can sometimes reassure, refuse to assess or undertake proper assessments, mislead, discharge and ignore Tribunal orders resulting in lost education for their children. The children are disabled by the lack of specialist provision so that they are often at the bottom of a mainstream class or in the bottom groups or sets regardless of their cognitive ability and potential. They are disabled by the type and speed of teaching in mainstream which does not take account of their needs. Giving full time teaching assistant support is not the answer for many children and can seriously affect the child's self-esteem and confidence. There seems to be little or no choice of provision and if it doesn't work the child is excluded. Time and pressure make the situation worse; specialists leave programmes for school staff to undertake instead of making them part of direct teaching or therapy. As a result, the children can become socially isolated and socially vulnerable. They are teased and bullied and gravitate towards the other problem children. If insufficient or inappropriate support is available, then mental health issues may result such as anxiety, despair, low self-esteem/self-image, phobias, depression, obsessions and fears, addictions and suicide.

This book is called 'Towards a positive future: Stories, ideas and inspiration from children with special educational needs, their families and professionals'. This chapter focuses on celebrating the strengths from the personal stories to give you ideas and inspiration for what we can do and what we know works to enable children and their families to achieve their potential and an ordinary life.

Clear description of the child's needs

When your child has additional needs which means that they need support at home, school or both, the first thing that you need is a clear and detailed description of those needs and what that means for the child's functioning, attainment and progress. This sounds straightforward. You hope that your GP, Health Visitor (HV) or pre-school teacher will either identify that there is a problem or listen to your concerns about your child's development and refer you for a single- or multidisciplinary assessment. You then hope that the assessment or assessments are carried out quickly by experienced doctors, therapists, psychologists or teachers, preferably in a local, convenient location on a mutually agreed day and time, and this does happen in some areas. You also hope that this leads to some form of early intervention or support. However, in some areas there may be staff vacancies, long waiting times, inexperienced professionals or a high turnover of staff which results in delay or inconsistency. This is where national and local support groups and charities and independent practitioners may be able to help. You will find a list of useful contacts in the Appendix.

Focus on abilities and strengths

Celebrate all achievements no matter how small, like Arthur's family who appreciate that he now likes eating out and good food, to the big achievements of students like Brandon who achieved 3 A levels, won Student of the Year, represented the Rotary Club in Europe and has gone to university. Caleb has passed Level 2 Motor Maintenance with distinction and is working in his own garage using his personal budget. Dexter is employed as a carpenter and lives independently with his girlfriend. Ernest has above average speech and language skills. Fatima achieved 5 A–C GCSEs. Gabriel always tries his best and has a positive attitude. Harvey enjoys fishing and sport and was on the gifted and talented register for public speaking. Ida works hard and enjoys many activities. She does ballet and has passed grade 5 piano with distinction. Jensen loves football, swimming and athletics, has 5 A–C grade GCSEs and is learning to drive. He is kind, caring and charming and hopes to go to college and work in construction. Keenan is happy and confident and achieved level 4 in his Science SAT. Lennox has taken on key roles in both the Physical Education and Design and Technology departments during his time in 6th form. He is part of the after-school cleaning team and has achieved a place at college to study furniture making and installation.

Milo is a sporty young man; he loves to play football and he swims for the District Swimming Club. He also loves cycling and hopes to complete his first triathlon. Nancy has learned to use the computer, can recognize 45 words and count up to 30. Orlando has begun communicating and has lost weight. He enjoys long walks and has a particular interest in birds.

This list could be describing any group of children in the land. You only know from reading their full personal stories in previous chapters that they have special educational needs. Their abilities and strengths enable us to be incredibly proud of this group of children and young people on an equal footing with all other parents and focuses us on their achievements as people first and on their impairments second. Never say never – encourage all children to meet and exceed all our expectations.

Productive activity promotes learning

By focusing on the interests of the children that we live and work with, the day at school and home can be filled with productive activity to promote learning. This will enhance their wellbeing and enable greater independence and vocational opportunities as they develop into adults. For this group long walks, appropriate exercise, music, art, sport, speech and drama and vocational skills are an important part of their curriculum in differing proportions. If a child is not able to take part in team sport due to their physical or medical needs, like Ernest, then rather than differentiating the sport curriculum and reinforcing for him that he is the worst in the class and different to his peers, it would be more appropriate to organize a productive and positive alternative activity during sport lessons focusing on his excellent speech and language skills or musical ability. He is unlikely to earn his future living playing sport but he may well become an actor or salesman.

Safe and secure physical environment

When choosing a school for your child, it is important that you are confident that the physical environment is safe and secure and appropriate to your child's needs. All schools should be accessible and be working towards enabling equality for all disabled people whether pupils, parents, visitors or staff. Making the adjustments necessary to improve any building by installing lifts, ramps, handrails and wide doorways, improving acoustics, ensuring different textures of flooring to identify different areas, keeping classrooms calm, low arousal environments with appropriate heating and lighting will enhance the learning experience for everyone. Equipment, and especially ICT equipment and resources, should also be available. Other features of schools that were successful in the personal stories were those that had small classes, a high adult:child ratio, good role models, other pupils with similar issues, a whole school approach and a sympathetic ethos. Again these features would enhance the education of all pupils in school.

Integrated therapy and teaching

If health, education and social care professionals were all based in schools so that speech and language therapists, occupational therapists, physiotherapists, psychotherapists and psychologists actively work alongside teachers and teaching assistants in the classroom so that therapy can inform teaching and teaching can inform therapy, it would become a normal part of every school day (Hatcher, 2011). This would enable the support, information, teaching and training from specialist teachers and therapists to be available for the student and their family to devise one plan which can then be implemented across the home and school settings. This integrated and consistent approach is far more effective, especially with the severe and complex needs of the children in our personal stories. For many, in order to achieve this they needed to attend specialist independent out-of-county residential schools. Of course pupils can follow programmes set by therapists and delivered by school staff, but the therapist needs to know the child individually in order to write a dynamic and meaningful programme and they need to know and demonstrate how it can be integrated into the timetable. It is not just what you do with a child that makes the difference but how you do it. The therapeutic relationship with the child and the relationships between professionals in schools are important to develop and they take time. Multi-agency planning was especially valued by the families in the featured stories around times of transition from one school to another, one class to another or indeed one phase of life to another. They also valued termly multi-agency meetings and close communication and liaison via home/school communication books, telephone or email.

Positive close relationship between school and home

The parents in our stories really appreciated having a close positive relationship with the school their child attended, other children and their families. We all need to view parents as key partners, offer family support and positive parenting training. This is especially important when the child has social, emotional and behavioural needs. The general strategies that help involved ignoring attention-seeking behaviour and rewarding positive behaviour immediately, sitting close to the class teacher and having an appropriate piece of equipment to fiddle with. These strategies would support all children and their families to improve the behaviour of all our children in the classroom.

Social care working in partnership with parents

A common thread is the lack of respite genuinely and consistently available to enable families to recharge their batteries and spend time parenting their other children as well as spending time as a family. Direct payments and personal budgets give that control back to the families and young people if there are support workers and link families available to employ in the same way that we employ child minders and babysitters for our other children. My concern at the moment, though, is the way these benefits are policed. I do not have any difficulty with providing the LA with receipts/invoices for all respite or activities commissioned but I do object to having to provide bank statements as well to corroborate the figures. The LA calculates how much respite is required through assessment. They cost that in order to pay the family. The family then provide a quarterly return with invoices/receipts to prove that they have spent the money on respite or approved activities. However, the family may be able to stretch the funding further by being creative with providers or may add to the funding in order to get more hours or buy in more expensive care. It is not in any family's interest to not spend the money on respite. If the LA does not trust you as a family to manage this budget they should not approve direct payments and should provide the respite directly instead. Demanding bank statements does not nurture an equal and trusting relationship with the family. The rest of the population are not asked to provide bank statements to prove how they spend their child benefit!

Availability of specialist programmes

Throughout the chapters some specialist programmes or approaches have been mentioned which families have found useful with their children. References to all these programmes and the websites where parents and professionals can get more information are in the Appendix. Many of these programmes and approaches are good practice and could be integrated into classrooms or offered by schools for all children. Examples of such programmes are 1, 2, 3 Magic, The Listening Programme, Social Communication Skills Programmes and Rebound Therapy.

Medication and nutrition

For some individuals medication is necessary or helpful to manage their needs, keep them well or minimize symptoms and this is always overseen by a doctor. For others, advice and support from a dietician or nutritional therapist and following a certain diet can help. This is true for many people with a wide variety of issues, not just those with special needs – diabetics and asthmatics, for example.

Access to specialist solicitors, representatives, expert witnesses and Tribunals when needed

This has been covered in the early chapters on the current SEN process and appeals and a list of useful organizations and solicitors can be found in the appendix.

Concluding remarks

We must recognize that it is our attitudes, beliefs and values that disable these youngsters and families rather than their impairments and prevent them from having the same ordinary educational and life chances as others in society. Individuals with special needs are all part of the rich diversity of our population. Let us hope that the imminent health, education and social care reforms will have listened to parents, professionals, pupils and teachers and undertake the radical changes that the system needs to ensure that all children are educated in the most appropriate place and in the most appropriate way for all their needs, including protecting and developing their self-esteem and confidence and enabling them to reach their potential, whatever that is.

11 Making it happen

Why

So now you've read the book, what are you going to do? When shortly after the 2010 general election the government started describing their vision for the future, the thing they called 'Big Society', people were deeply sceptical; and rightly so, for we'd endured some 40 years of 'top down' government. People didn't necessarily like being told what was best for them, but at least they knew where they stood.

Then, in the summer of 2011, a number of factors transformed the 'Big Society' rhetoric into the Big Reality. It started with the *News of the World* and the phone hacking scandal. Politicians eager to remain squeaky clean after the earlier parliamentary expenses scandal now found themselves smeared once more; tarnished and blotted and transparently vulnerable, frail and in some cases greedy. Rioting, looting, appalling street crime and murder pulled down the Big Society dream. People were not starving, or particularly desperate. They simply saw the opportunity to update their phone, grab the latest flat screen TV or just stock up on booze for a party, all for free. Volunteering and selfless giving was the government's hope for us. Instead, many chose publicly and brutally to demonstrate materialism and greed. It would be fitting to find some of the 2011 rioters sharing cells with disgraced city bankers. In fact, the disgrace is that this is possible. It's no wonder few people bother to vote. So what is the Big Reality we're left with?

To put it crudely, we can no longer kid ourselves that quarts can be extracted from pint pots. Government borrowing has grown, maintaining the illusion that the impossible is achievable. The US has chosen to keep borrowing; and denial always ends in tears. Do we really want to end up like them? We have an ageing population, low economic growth and too many people who expect stuff to just happen when they need it.

We must now focus on this new, stark future. The underlying challenges arenot going to go away; we all need to confront them. Leaving it to government, local authorities, the NHS or Job Centre Plus has not delivered what we need. It has simply hidden the issues behind walls of bureaucracy, a plethora of processes at vast public expense.

But you are not a politician, or a rioter. Instead you are an honest, law-abiding citizen. What unites you with other readers is your interest in 'special educational needs'. You might be a parent, determined to secure the best start in life for your child, or a teacher or perhaps a health professional, struggling to deliver what you know is needed when the time and money to do this just isn't there.

What

It may have always been up to you to make things happen. Now that's truer than ever before.

In fact, the whole rationale behind current government policy is to empower you as an individual to take control of your own destiny. In theory, personal budgets, the devolution of accountability and the dissolution of state monopoly should stimulate a vibrant, dynamic, marketed social economy. In reality, they're creating confusion and a vacuum into which you may well currently feel sucked. So you need to take control.

First, you need to set aside past prejudices, perceptions and, at times, practices. The Big Reality we now face means you need to think differently. Do this and you'll be amongst the first to benefit from tomorrow's new order. Here are some things to reflect on:

- Stop blaming 'them' for our societal ills. You are society; you face the opportunity and you need to speak up so that others will follow.
- Start with the facts and focus people's minds on the simple fact that government spending comes from our pockets; the more we do ourselves, the less tax we will need to pay and the better services we get.
- Economic growth is not a panacea, except perhaps in sectors that reduce material consumption. SEN is not about materialism, but potential.
- We cannot go back, so there's no point in complaining about what's already taken place.
- You can't change the world on your own, but you do need to be the first to step forward and make a start.

It's a case of recognizing, then realizing, that you hold the key that can unlock the change you want to see.

Who

You can do something. Perhaps not much, and each of you might do slightly different things, but if you all act, big things will happen. It's how revolutions are won.

The SEN landscape is ripe for revolution. Statementing, funding, referral, support and every other aspect of the process is clunky, unwieldy and, too often, puts paperwork ahead of people. But it's changing.

Parents can create their own SEN schools under the Free School banner. Health professionals can be supported into social enterprise, escaping the bureaucracy of the NHS. Parents are increasingly well informed and thus are better able to say 'No' to what feels inadequate and to find new ways to secure the support their youngsters need.

But the common factor in all of this is you. You have to be willing to take some modest risks and actually do something. Let me give you an odd example. Trevor Baylis invented the wind-up radio. He did this in response to seeing a TV programme that reported the challenges faced by organizations trying to communicate positive public health information in sub-Saharan Africa. The problem was that, because of intermittent power supply, people could not listen to radio.

Baylis got off his sofa, walked through to his workshop and got started. Yes, he was an engineer but, more important than that, he felt motivated to act. He was by no means the best qualified person to make this invention. He just went and did it.

Don't doubt your own ability or qualification to prompt or create the change you want to see. The most important thing is that you want to do it, understand why it's important and have the passion and drive that only come from personal experience.

How

How you do stuff depends a lot on what you want to do. If you're a parent, frustrated by the lack of support, you might start an action group, lobby or simply find a way to pay. Professionals, on the other hand, are more likely to start their own enterprise.

Many people find it restricting and frustrating when an organizational structure prevents them from working in the way they feel best suits them and their client group. The dramatic changes we are seeing in the health, education and social care worlds make it easier than ever before for you to change the way things are done. It would be impossible to tell you exactly what's going to work for you.

However, there are some basic principles that will apply to anyone involved with SEN who wants to change things. Here they are.

- Develop a clear vision of what it is you want to change and be sure you fully understand why.
- Share your vision with others and be prepared to adapt if they surprise you and don't agree.
- Remember that it's way easier to take lots of small steps than a few giant leaps.
- Don't doubt your ability or conviction – even if others do. Just focus and go for it.
- Remember that people only do things when they can see a clear benefit to them – do not rely on goodwill or altruism.
- There's little new. Take time to find out what's already been done elsewhere and copy what worked.

Concluding remarks

Now you're at the end of this book, you face some very simple choices. If you were moved by the stories and inspired by how parents and professionals have already made a difference, then it's time you got off the chair and made a start too.

Appendix

Useful contacts

National support groups and charities

This list is not exhaustive but it is somewhere to start to find the UK website links for national charities and support groups which may point you in the right direction. It is difficult to find the right organization if you don't know exactly what you are looking for. It also assumes that you have access to or can get access to a computer either at home or via your local library. Professionals may assume you know where to go to get information if you are given a medical diagnosis or label. Please don't assume and please do give your families as much information as possible particularly about local contacts, networks and support groups. Also do offer to search for them or enable them to have access to a computer if needed.

The Association for Rehabilitation of Communication and Oral Skills (ARCOS) – www.arcos.org.uk – is a national charity that works with children and adults who have communication and eating (swallowing) difficulties, their families, carers and others involved. ARCOS provides information, advice, practical help, specialist therapy, training and other services not readily available elsewhere.

Association for All Speech Impaired Children (AFASIC) – www.afasicengland.org.uk – supports parents and carers of children with speech and language impairments.

The Association of Spina Bifida and Hydrocephalus (ASBAH) – www.asbah.org – is a UK-registered charity providing information and advice about spina bifida and hydrocephalus.

National Autistic Society (NAS) – www.autism.org.uk – is the leading UK charity for people with autism (including Asperger syndrome) and their families. They provide information, support and pioneering services, and campaign for a better world for people with autism.

The British Institute for Brain Injured Children – www.bibic.org.uk – is a registered charity encouraging home-based therapy to help children variously diagnosed as having autism, autistic tendencies and brain damage.

Cerebra –www.cerebra.org.uk – is a unique charity set up to help improve the lives of children with brain-related conditions through research, education and directly supporting the children and their carers.

The Challenging Behaviour Foundation – www.thecbf.org.uk – wants to see children and adults with severe learning disabilities, who are described as having challenging behaviour, having the same life opportunities as everyone else, including home life, education, employment and leisure.

Child Brain Injury Trust (CBIT) – www.childbraininjurytrust.org.uk – helps children, young people, their families and professionals to come to terms with what has happened and how to deal with the uncertainty that the future holds.

Cleft Lip and Palate Association – www.clapa.com – is the representative organization for all people with and affected by cleft lip and/or palate in the UK.

Contact-a-family (CAF) – www.cafamily.org.uk – is a national support group for the families of those with special needs.

Dyslexia Action – www.dyslexiaaction.org.uk – is the biggest dyslexia charity in the UK. It provides a wide range of services to people of all ages who have dyslexia and struggle with literacy.

CReSTeD – www.crested.org.uk - is a Register that helps children with specific learning difficulties (dyslexia) choose schools. All schools included in the Register are visited regularly to ensure they continue to meet the criteria set by CReSTeD.

Down's Syndrome Association – www.downs-syndrome.org.uk – helps people with Down's syndrome to live full and rewarding lives.

Dyspraxia Foundation – www.dyspraxiafoundation.org.uk – supports individuals and families affected by developmental dyspraxia through books, suggestions, a teen newsletter, and an adult support group.

Family Action – www.family-action.org.uk – is a charity which has been a leading provider of services to disadvantaged and socially isolated families since its foundation in 1869. They work with over 45,000 children and families a year by providing practical, emotional and financial support through over 100 services based in communities across England. A further 150,000 people benefit from their educational grants and information service. They tackle some of the most complex and difficult issues facing families today – including domestic abuse, mental health problems, learning disabilities and severe financial hardship as these issues have a huge impact on the wellbeing and development of children; and on the ability of parents and carers to make a positive contribution to their community. They work with whole families to help them find solutions to problems, no matter how difficult, so that they become safer, stronger and more optimistic about their future

ICAN – www.ican.org.uk – is a charity that supports children with speech, language and communication difficulties.

Mencap – www.mencap.org.uk – is the voice of learning disability.

The National Attention Deficit Disorder Information and Support Service – www.addiss.co.uk

National Deaf Children's Society (NDCS) – www.ndcs.org.uk – their mission is to remove the barriers to the achievement of deaf children around the world.

RNIB – www.rnib.org.uk – offers support and advice to blind and partially sighted people in the UK, helping people who have lost their sight to find their lives again.

Scope – www.scope.org.uk – is a charity that supports physically disabled people with cerebral palsy and their families.

Signature – www.signature.org.uk – promotes excellence in communication with deaf and deafblind people.

Symbol – www.symboluk.co.uk – provides specialist speech and language therapy consultation and services to children and adults with special needs who experience learning and social needs, including those with Downs Syndrome.

www.talkingpoint.org.uk – is a website that provides information on children's communication.

Young Minds – www.youngminds.org.uk – is a UK charity concerned with the mental health and well being of our young people and their families

Specialist programmes, approaches and services

www.alertprogram.com

www.bobath.org.uk

www.braingym.org.uk

www.britishsignlanguage.com

www.bsmt.org

www.conductive-education.org.uk

www.hanen.org

www.intensiveinteraction.co.uk

www.thelisteningproramme.com

www.makaton.org

www.pgss.org

www.pecs.org.uk

www.reboundtherapy.org

www.wendyrinaldi.com

www.autismtreatmentcenter.org

www.teacch.com

www.omegaAIT.com

www.alexkelly.biz

www.wordswell.co.uk

www.speechandlanguage-therapy.com

Organizations for professionals and to help parents find professionals

www.helpwithtalking.com

www.bps.org.uk

www.childpsychotherapy.org.uk

www.aep.org.uk

www.bacp.co.uk

www.baat.org

www.badth.org.uk

www.baot.org.uk

www.bapt.info

www.batod.org.uk

www.csp.org.uk

www.hpc-uk.org

www.isc.co.uk

www.rcslt.org

www.awcebd,co.uk

www.nasen.org.uk

www.thecommunicationtrust.org.uk

www.comunicationsforum.org.uk

Specialist schools

A list of all schools for special needs – state and independent – can be found in the Gabbitas Guide – www.gabbitas.co.uk. SCOPE, ICAN and the NAS all run their own specialist schools. This is a list of specialist schools I have visited who are successful at educating children with SEN. Please see their own websites for more details.

Eagle House School – www.eaglehouseschool.com
Cruckton Hall School – www.cruckton.com
St David's College – www.stdavidscollege.co.uk
Mary Hare School – www.maryhare.org.uk
Priors Court School – www.priorscourt.org.uk
St Christopher's School, Bristol – www.st-christophers.bristol.sch.uk
Alderwasley Hall School – www.alderwasleyhall.com
Stanbridge Earls – www.stanbridgeearls.co.uk
St Catherine's School – www.stcatherines.org.uk
Blossom House School – www.blossomhouseschool.co.uk
Centre Academy – www.centreacademylondon.eu
Tree House – www.treehouseschool.org.uk
Sutherland House School – www.sutherlandhouse.org.uk
Shapwick School – www.shapwickschool.com
Maple Hayes Hall School – www.dyslexia.gb.com
The Link School – www.link-sec.sutton.sch.uk
Moor House School – www.moorhouse.surrey.sch.uk
More House School – www.morehouseschool.com
St Mary's Wrestwood Children's Trust – www.st-marys.bexhill.sch.uk
St John's Catholic School for the Deaf – www.stjohns.org.uk
Gretton School – www.grettonschool.com

Other specialist schools are run by

Priory Education Services – www.priorygroup.com
Hesley Group – www.hesleygroup.co.uk
Cambian – www.cambiangroup.com

Acorn Care – www.acorncare.co.uk

Piscari – www.piscari.com

Some support organizations providing lay representation/educational advocacy

Education Advocacy (EA) – www.educationadvocacy.co.uk

Advocacy Services and Special Education Training (ASSET) is a small independent charity which provides information and advice about education to parents/carers of children with special educational needs who live in England – www.asset-gb.org

AM Phillips Education Law Ltd – www.amphillips.co.uk

SOS!SEN – www.sossen.org.uk

Independent Panel for Special Educational Advice (IPSEA) – www.ipsea.org.uk -

Network 81 – www.network81.org

Office for Advice, Assistance, Support and Information on Special Needs – www.oaasis.co.uk – provide an information service for parents and professionals, including factsheets available to download.

Some specialist education law solicitors

Anthony Collins – www.anthonycollins.com

Children's Legal Centre – www.childrenslegalcentre.com

Douglas Silas – www.specialeducationalneeds.co.uk

MG Law Ltd – www.maxwellgillott.com

Christopher Davidson – www.cdlaw.co.uk

Langley Wellington – www.langleywellington.co.uk

Fisher Meredith – www.fishermeredith.co.uk

Other useful websites

Bond Solon – www.bondsolon.com – the medico-legal training consultancy

Expert Witness Institute – www.ewi.org.uk

Robert Ashton – www.robertashton.co.uk

SEN Magazine – www.senmagazine.co.uk

Bangor University – www.bangor.ac.uk

University of Wales – www.newport.ac.uk

Local Government Ombudsman – www.lgo.org.uk

References and suggested reading

Andron, L. (2001) *Our Journey Through High Functioning Autism & Asperger Syndrome.* London: Jessica Kingsley Publishing.

Ashton, R. (2008) *I Know Someone Like That. One Man's Search for Normal in Norfolk.* Turnpike Farm.

Ashton, R. (2010) *How to be a Social Entrepreneur: Make Money and Change the World.* Chichester: Capstone.

Attwood, T. (2006) *A Complete Guide to Asperger Syndrome.* London: Jessica Kingsley Publishers.

Barnes, C. (2004) Disability, disability studies and the academy. In J. Swain, S. French, C., Barnes & C. Thomas (Eds) *Disabling Barriers, Enabling Environments.* London: Sage.

Barnes, C. (2008) Generating change: Disability, culture and art. *Journal of Disability and International Development, 1,* 4–13.

Barton, L. (2004) The disability movement: Some observations. In J. Swain, S. French, C., Barnes & C. Thomas (Eds) *Disabling Barriers, Enabling Environments.* London: Sage.

Beardon, L. & Edmonds, G. 2007 ASPECT consultancy report. www.shu.ac.uk/theautismcentre

The Bercow Report (2008) *A Review of Services for Children and Young People (0–19) with Speech, Language and Communication Needs.* London: HMSO.

Birnbaum, R. (2010) *Choosing a School for a Child with Special Needs.* London: Jessica Kingsley Publishing.

Bond, C., Solon, M. & Harper, P. (1999) *The Expert Witness in Court. A Practical Guide.* Crayford: Shaw and Sons.

Botting, N., Faragher, B., Simkin, Z., Knox, E. & Conti-Ramsden, G. (2001) Predicting Pathways of Specific Language Impairment: What Differentiates Good and Poor Outcome? *Journal of Child Psychology and Psychiatry and Allied Disciplines, 42(8),* 1013–1020.

Botting, N. & Conti-Ramsden, G. (2000) Social and behavioural difficulties in children with language impairment. *Child Language Teaching and Therapy, 16(2),* 105–120.

Cameron, C. (2008) Further towards an Affirmative Model. In T. Campbell et al. (Eds) *Disability Studies. Emerging Insights and Perspectives.* Leeds: The Disability Press.

Cameron, C. (2011) Not our problem. Disability as role. In press.

Conti-Ramsden, G., Botting, N., Simkin, Z. & Knox, E. (2001) Follow-up of children attending infant language units: Outcomes at 11 years of age. *International Journal of Language and Communication Disorders, 36*, 207–219.

Conti-Ramsden, G. & Botting, N. (2008) Emotional health in adolescents with and without a history of specific language impairment (SLI). *Journal of Child Psychology and Psychiatry, 49*, 516–525.

Conti-Ramsden, G., Botting, N., Knox, E.,& Simkin, Z. (2002). Different school placements following language unit attendance: Which factors affect langage outcome? *International Journal of Language & Communication Disorders, 37(2)*, 185–195.

Conti-Ramsden, G., Knox, E., Botting, N. & Simkin, Z. (2002) Educational placements and National Curriculum Key Stage 2 test outcomes of children with a history of specific language impairment. *British Journal of Special Education, 29(2)*, 76–82.

Conti-Ramsden, G., Durkin, K., Simkin, Z. & Knox, E. (2009) Specific language impairment and school outcomes. I: Identifying and explaining variability at the end of compulsory education. *International Journal of Language & Communication Disorders, 44(1)*, 15–35.

Corker, M. & Shakespeare, T. (Eds) (2002) *Embodying Disability Theory. Disability Postmodernism*. London/NY: Continuum.

Crow, L. (1996) Including all of our lives: Renewing the Social Model of Disability. In J. Morris (Ed.) *Encounters with Strangers*. London: The Women's Press.

Disability Discrimination Act 1995. https://www.ehrc.gov

Durkin, K., Simkin, Z., Knox, E. & Conti-Ramsden, G. (2009) Specific language impairment and school outcomes. II: Educational context, student satisfaction, and post-compulsory progress. *International Journal of Language & Communication Disorders, 44(1)*, 36–55.

Easton, C, Sheach, S. & Easton, S. (1997) Teaching vocabulary to children with word finding difficulties using a combined semantic and phonological approach: an efficacy study. *Child Language Teaching and Therapy, 13(2)*, 125–142.

Equality Act 2010. https://www.ehrc.gov

Edelman, M. (2001) Social movements: Changing paradigms and forms of politics. *Annual Review of Anthropology, 30*, 285–317.

Eldevik, S., Hastings, R.P., Hughes, J.C., Jahr, E., Eikeseth, S. & Cross, S. (2009) Meta-analysis of Early Intensive Behavioural Intervention for Children with Autism. *Journal of Clinical Child and Adolescent Psychology, 38*, 439–450.

Goffman, G. (1961) *Asylums: Essays on the Social Situation of Mental Patients and Other Inmates*. New York: Doubleday.

Goodley, D. (2010). *Disability Studies. An Interdisciplinary Introduction*. London: Sage.

Goodley, D. & Runswick-Cole, K. (2011). The violence of disablism. *Sociology of Health and Illness, 33(4)*, 602–617.

Haller, B., Dorries, B. & Rahn, J. (2006) Media labelling versus the US disability community identity: A study of shifting cultural language. *Disability and Society, 21(1)*, 61–75.

Hannaford, C. (1995) *Smart Moves. Why Learning Is Not All In Your Head*. Arlington, VA: Great Ocean Publishers.

Hatcher, C. (2011) *Making Collaborative Practice Work. A Model for Teachers and SLTs*. Guildford: J & R Press Ltd.

Hayward, D., Eikeseth, S., Gale, C. & Morgan, S. (2009) Assessing progress during treatment for young children with autism receiving intensive behavioural interventions. *Autism, 13(6)*, 613–633.

Hirschman, M. (2000) Language repair via metalinguistic means. *International Journal of Language and Communication Disorders, 35(2)*, 251–268.

Hoong-Sin, C. & Fong, J. (2008) The impact of regulatory fitness requirements on disabled social work students. *British Journal of Social Work on Line*, 31 May, 1–22.

Ireland, Jane L. (2008) Psychologists as witnesses: Background and good practice in the delivery of evidence. *Educational Psychology in Practice, 24(2)*, 115–127.

Jackson, L. (2002) *Freaks, Geeks and Asperger Syndrome. A User Guide to Adolescence*. London: Jessica Kingsley Publishing.

Johnson, M. & Wintgens, A (2001) *The Selective Mutism Resource Manual*. Milton Keynes: Speechmark.

Johnson, M. & Wintgens, A. (2001) *The Selective Mutism Resource Manual*. Milton Keynes: Speechmark Publishing Ltd.

Kuppers, P. (2002) Image politics, without the real: Simulacra, dandyism and disability fashion. In M. Corker & T. Shakespeare (Eds) E*mbodying Disability Theory. Disability Postmodernism*, pp184–197. London: Continuum.

Kuppers, P. (2003) D*isability and Contemporary Performance. Bodies on the Edge*. London: Routledge.

Lamb Inquiry (2009) *Special Educational Needs and Parental Confidence*. London: HMSO.

Law, J. et al. (2000) Provision for children's speech and language needs in England and Wales: Facilitating communication between education and health services. DfES research report 239. London: HMSO.

Law, J., Garrett, Z. & Nye, C. (2003) SLT interventions for children with primary speech and language delay or disorder. *Cochrane Database of Systematic Reviews*, Issue 3. Art. No.: CD004110. DOI: 10.1002/14651858.CD004110

Law, J., Lindsay, G., Peacey, N., Gascoigne, M., Soloff, N., Radford, J., Band, S. & Fitzgerald, L. (2000) *Provision for Children with Speech and Language Needs in En,gland and Wales: Facilitating Communication Between Education and Health Service*. London: DfES Publications http://www.dfes.gov.uk/research/

Locke, A., Ginsborg, J. & Peers, I. (2002) Development and disadvantage: Implications for early years. *Journal of Language Communication Disorders, 37(1)*, 3–15.

Lovaaas, O.I. (1987) Behavioral treatment and normal educational and intellectual functioning in young autistic children. *Journal of Consulting Clinical Psychology, 55(1),* 3–9.

Madriaga, M., Goodley, D., Hodge, N. & Martin, N. (2008) Experiences and identities of UK students with Asperger syndrome. www.heacademy.ac.uk/events/detail.researchseminar

Martin, N. (2008) REAL services to assist university students who have Asperger syndrome. NADP Technical briefing 2008/4

Martin, N. (2010) A preliminary study of disability themes in the Edinburgh fringe festival. *Disability and Society, 25(5),* 539–549.

Martin, N. & Hendrickx, S (2011) Insights into intimacy from people with Asperger syndrome and their partners. *Good Autism Practice, 12(10),* 26–33.

Mallett, R. (in press) Claiming comedic immunity: Or, what do you get when you cross contemporary British comedy with disability. *Review of Disability Studies.*

May, H. & Bridger, K. (2010) *Developing and Embedding Inclusive Policy and Practice in Higher Education.* York: The Higher Education Academy.

McRuer, R. (2003) As good as it gets: Queer theory and critical disability. *GLQ: A Journal of Lesbian and Gay Studies, (9.1–2),* 79–105.

McRuer, R. (2008) *Crip Theory. Cultural Signs of Queerness and Disability.* New York: New York University Press.

Middleton, J.A. (2001) Brain injury in children and adolescents. *Advances in Psychiatric Treatment, 7,* 257–265.

Murphy, F. (2008) The clinical experience of dyslexic healthcare students. www.sciencedirect.com/science

Nightingale, C. (2007) *Disabled Staff in Adult and Continuing Education.* Leicester: NIACE.

Oliver, M. (2009) *Understanding Disability, from Theory to Practice,* 2nd ed. Basingstoke: Palgrave Macmillan.

Peer, L. & Reid, G. (2011) *Special Educational Needs. A Guide for Inclusiv Practice.* London: Sage Publications.

Peters, S. (2000). Is there a disability culture? A syncretisation of three possible world views. *Disability and Society, 15(4),* 583–601.

Petersen, L. & Lewis, P. (2004) *Stop, Think, Do Social Skills Training: Supplement for Middle Years of Schooling Ages.* Australian Centre for Education.

Phelan, T. (2003) *1-2-3 Magic.* Glen Ellyn, IL: Child Management Inc.

Picard, M. & Bradley, J.S. (2001) Revisiting speech interference in classrooms. *Audiology, 40(5),* 221–244.

Reid, J., Millar, S., Tait, L., Donaldson, M., Dean, E.C., Thomson, G.O.B. & Grieve, R. (1996) Pupils with special educational needs: The role of SLTs. *Interchange, (43).*

Richards, R. (2008) Writing the othered self. Autoethnography and the problem of objectification in writing about disability and illness. *The Journal of Qualitative Health Research, 18(12),* 1717–1728.

Rogers, S.J. & Vismara, L.A. (2008) Evidence-based comprehensive treatments for early autism. *Journal of Clinical Child and Adolescent Psychology, 37,* 8–38.

The Rose Report (2009) *Independent Review of the Primary Curriculum.* London: HMSO.

Row, S. (2005) *Surviving the Special Educational Needs System. How to be a Velvet Bulldozer.* London: Jessica Kingsley Publishing.

Sandahl, C. (2008) Why disability identity matters: From dramaturgy to casting in John Belluso's Pyretown. *Text and Performance Quarterly, 28(1–2),* 225–241.

Shakespeare, T. (1999) Joking a part. *Body and Society, 5(4),* 47–52.

Shakespeare, T. (2006) *Disability Rights and Wrong.* London: Routledge.

Shaw, J. (2002) *I'm Not Naughty – I'm Autistic. Jody's Journey.* London: Jessica Kingsley Publishing.

Silvers, A. (2002) The crooked timber of humanity: Disability, ideology, aesthetic. In M. Corker & T. Shakespeare (Eds) *Embodying Disability Theory. Disability and Postmodernism,* pp 228–244. London: Continuum.

Snowling, Margaret J. & Hayiou-Thomas, Marianna E. (2006) The dyslexia spectrum: Continuities between reading, speech, and language impairments. *Topics in Language Disorders, 26(2),* 110–126.

Tomblin, J.B., Records, N.L. et al. (1997) Prevalence of specific language impairment in kindergarten children. *Journal of Speech, Language, and Hearing Research, 40(6),* 1245–1260.

Valentine, J. 2002. Naming and narrating disability in Japan. In M. Corker & T. Shakespeare (Eds) *Embodying Disability Theory. Disability and Postmodernism,* pp 213–227. London/NY: Continuum.

Warnock, M. & Norwich, B. (2010) *Special Educational Needs. A New Look.* London: Continuum International Publishing Group.

Wells, J. (2006) *Touch and Go Joe. An Adolescent's Experience of OCD.* London: Jessica Kingsley Publishers.

Glossary

ABA	Applied Behavioural Analysis
ADDISS	Attention Deficit Disorder Information and Support Service
ADD	Attention Deficit Disorder
ADHD	Attention Deficit Hyperactivity Disorder
AFASIC	Association for All Speech Impaired Children
AS	Asperger Syndrome
ASC	Autistic Spectrum Condition
ASLTIP	Association of Speech and Language Therapists in Independent Practice
BCBA	Board Certified Behaviour Analyst
BESC	Behavioural Emotional and Social Condition
BESD	Behavioural Emotional and Social Disability
BSL	British Sign Language
CAMHS	Child and Adolescent Mental Health Service
CDC	Child Development Centre
DIY	Do It Yourself
DSM-V	Diagnostic and Statistical Manual of Mental Disorders, Fifth Edition

DVD	Digital Versatile Disc
EBD	Emotional and Behavioural Disability
EIBI	Early Intensive Behavioural Intervention
EP	Educational Psychologist
GCSE	General Certificate of Secondary Education
GP	General Practitioner
IBI	Intensive Behavioural Intervention
ICT	Information and Communication Technology
IEP	Individual Education Plan
IPSEA	Independent Panel for Special Educational Advice
LA	Local Authority
LEA	Local Education Authority
LSA	Learning Support Assistant
MLD	Moderate Learning Disability
MOJ	Ministry of Justice
NAS	National Autistic Society
NHS	National Health Service
NLP	Neuro-Linguistic Programming
NVQ	National Vocational Qualification
ODD	Oppositional Defiant Disorder
OT	Occupational Therapy

PECS	Picture Exchange Communication System
RCSLT	Royal College of Speech and Language Therapists
SALT	Speech and Language Therapist
SAT	Standard Attainment Test
SEN	Special Educational Needs
SENCO	Special Educational Needs Coordinator
SENDIST	Special Educational Needs and Disability Tribunal
SLCN	Speech Language and Communication Needs
SPELL	Structure, Positive approaches and expectations, Empathy, Low arousal and Links
SpLD	Specific Learning Disability
SLD	Severe Learning Disability
SLT	Speech and Language Therapist
SSRI	Selective Serotonin Reuptake Inhibitor
TA	Teaching Assistant
TEACCH	**T**reatment and **E**ducation of **A**utistic and **C**ommunication related handicapped **CH**ildren
TV	Television
UK	United Kingdom
VB	Verbal Behaviour